MATERIA MEDICA

OF

SEXUAL DISORDERS

By

Nikunj Trivedi

Previously Published Books by Dr. Nikunj

1. Homeopathy for Sexual disorders
(Repertory of Infertility)

2. Sperm Abnormality & Homeopathy
(Under publication with IBPS)

Note from the Author:

Any information given in this book is not intended to be taken as a replacement for medical advice. It is only for reference purpose. This book provides unique comparative study of the drug picture and disease picture.

Any person with a condition requiring medical attention should consult qualified Homeopath or Medical practitioner.

Order this book online at www.trafford.com
or email orders@trafford.com

Most Trafford titles are also available at major online book retailers.

Author Credits: Amita Trivedi / Arti Trivedi
1st Edition: 2010

Printed in the United States of America.

ISBN: 978-1-4269-5826-7 (sc)

Trafford rev. 02/18/2011

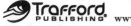 www.trafford.com

North America & international
toll-free: 1 888 232 4444 (USA & Canada)
phone: 250 383 6864 ♦ fax: 812 355 4082

Dedication

To,
My all valued patients who put their
Faith
In
Homeopathy

Special thanks to my dearest son, Parth for his valuable inputs during the course of preparation of this book.

Contents

Preface

This book is intended to cover the "Human Sexual Disorders" in a comprehensive and therapeutic manner for explanation and remedial indication of Materia –Medica.

The aim of the book is to encourage homeopathic students and practitioners to learn and understand about the use of clinical Homeopathy with a complexity of diseases, in a simplified way. This book will aid them in building successful scientific evidence based clinical applications of Materia Medica.The idea for this book dawned after coming across many clinical conditions during my training and working in Obstetric and Gynaecology department. Here, I have tried to portray the essential inter-relationships between the disease and drug picture in a comparative manner to retain every valuable morsel of knowledge.

This book is aimed at those wanting to practice clinical homeopathy in Reproductive Disorders, where prolonged use of conventional medicine having a serious outbreak of side effects. This book could be used as a quick guide to select a remedy for reproductive disorders.

Undoubtedly, vast clinical experience and all time medical supervision are always essential to practice Gynaecological conditions for those who understand the pathology of the disease. I am sure this book will bring a new revolution in Homeopathic world for new generation of Homeopaths.

About book

This Book is an effort to separate, convert and compare the symptoms narrated in Boericke's Materia-Medica in more appropriate scientific and in clinical forms. The book promises to prove useful to both students and experienced homeopaths. It is an attempt to familiarize the reader, to symptom conversion and the clinical aspects of Materia Medica.

Nikunj's deep insights have profoundly influenced the way many homeopaths want to practice today. Nikunj is particularly keen on encouraging his colleagues and juniors to search for the central disturbance within the individual due to psycho-somatic factors, which are expanding the concept and spectrum of miasmatic classification reflecting on reproductive derangement.

This well written and well presented book contains the clinical application of "the well -known verified characteristic symptoms of all our medicines" as said by William Boericke, in his Materia Medica.

About Author

Nikunj Trivedi has been in clinical practice since 1980. Nikunj has practiced clinical Homeopathy in India until 2004; however he is currently based in the United Kingdom. Nikunj has successfully treated over 30,000 patients from all over the world and is actively providing homeopathic training to prospective students.

Nikunj's interest lies in developing clinical applications of homeopathy in reproductive disorders. Working intensively in Gynaecology and Obstetrics department, he has developed comparative and clinical skill to understand clinical applications of homeopathic Materia- Medica. This inspired him to explore the latent potential of Homeopathy in disorders where conventional medicine has its own limitations.

Nikunj is committed to individuality, simplicity, clarity and perfection. He enjoys reading, writing poetry, listening music and spending quality time with his family.

Introduction

Alphabetical index

Introduction
Basics of Male Reproductive System

It is vital to understand the basic anatomy and physiology of male reproductive organs, which comprises of Testes, Epididymis, Seminal Vesicles and Prostate, Prostatic Urethra and Penis. As shown in
Figure 1.

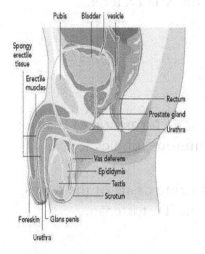

Figure 1 showing the male reproductive system (http://nursingcrib.com/functions-of-the-male-reproductive-

TESTES

- Two flat oval bodies.
- One on each side.
- Hanging outside the body in a sac called – "Scrotum".
- It is covered tough, compact fibrous capsule called- Tunica Albugenia.
- From Tunica Albugenia, traebecule descend and divide the testes in to a number of pyramidal lobules.
- These lobules are filled up with a convoluted Seminiferous Tubules.

- Each seminiferous tubule is 500mm long.
  Several seminiferous tubules are uniting to form a Straight Tubules.
- Several straight tubules unite to form a Rete Testes.
- These all joins to form a Vasa Efferentia.
- It finally combines to form the duct of Epididymis.
- The whole epididymis having a 6 meters long convoluted tubule which is very long and remaining coiled up together at the back of the testes and ultimately continued as the Vas Deferens.

Function of testes

1. **Spermatogenesis:**
   Spermatogenesis, the process of formation of mature sperm, takes place in seminiferous tubules.
2. **Testosterone secretion:**
   Interstitial cells are the endocrine tissue of the testes, which synthesise the hormone Testosterone.

What is testosterone?

Interstitial cells of Leydig are stimulated by the gonadotrophins. The chief products which are secreted in to the spermatic venous blood of adult testes are testosterone and very small quantity of dehydroepiandrosterone. Testosterone (a steroid hormone secreted by the testes), is a male sex hormone. It belongs to the broad group of androgens.

Functions of testosterone (androgen)

1. **Growth and development of male sex organs**
   - Like the seminal vesicles, prostate, epididymis, vas deferens, penis etc.
   - Maintenance of the morphologic and functional activity of seminal vesicles.
   - Enlargement of seminal vesicles to enable fructose secretion

2. **Development of male secondary sex characters**
   - Development of male pattern of body hair distribution and masculine voice
   - Activity and emotional picture of the male
   - Increasing the life-span and fertilising power of spermatozoa.

3. **Muscular development**
   - Testosterone has protein anabolic property, thus it aids in increasing the bone matrix and deposition of calcium salts, therefore allowing muscular development
   - It also enhances the closure of epiphysis of long bones and thus arrests the growth.

4. **Positive nitrogen balance**
   - It increases the passage of Amino acids insides the cell and improves and maintains the Positive Nitrogen Balance by nitrogen retaining effect.

5. **Basal metabolic rate (BMR)**
   - Testosterone increases the BMR. This effect might also be secondary to the protein anabolic property of the hormone.

6. **Effect on Red Blood Cells (R.B.C.)**
   - The higher total R.B.C. in males compared to females is attributed to the effects of testosterone.
7. **Effects on water and mineral metabolism**
   - Testosterone causes retention of
     - Sodium
     - Potassium
     - Calcium and
     - Phosphate and water also to some extent.
8. **Male psycho-sexual behaviour**
   - Testosterone is responsible for development of the male psycho-sexual behavioural pattern.

9. **Leutinising hormone (LH) inhibition**
   - Testosterone has an inhibitory effect on LH secretion by the pituitary gland.

EPIDIDYMIS
- Epididymis has a Pseudo stratified epithelium with tall columnar cells and basal cells.
- The surface cells contain the secretary granules.
- The epididymis acts as a 'store house' of spermatozoa, until ejaculation occurs.
- Even if an ejaculation does not take place, the spermatozoa are produced.
- The un-ejaculated spermatozoa are re-absorbed in Vas Deference.

SEMINAL VESICLE

The vas deference is joined by the duct of the seminal vesicle which is a musculo-glandular sac to form the ejaculatory duct. The ejaculatory duct opens in to prostatic urethra. The secretion of the prostate and seminal vesicles makes up a considerable part of the semen.

The seminal vesicle **does not** store spermatozoa. It acts an 'activator' for the sperms.

The secretion of seminal vesicles contains -
1. Fructose
2. Ascorbic acid
3. Citric acid
4. Inorganic phosphorous
5. Acid soluble phosphorous
6. Electrolytes
7. Protein
8. Ergothioneine
9. Enzymes like Creatine Phosphokinase (CPK)

The secretion of prostate contains -
1. Spermine
2. Citric acid
3. Cholesterol
4. Phospholipids
5. Fibrinolysin
6. Fibrinogenase

All these have important functions for the nourishments of the sperms. The prostate contributes about 20% of total volume of Human Semen.

SEMEN

Semen is an organic fluid that usually contains spermatozoa. It is secreted by the gonads (sexual glands) and other sexual organs of male.

Semen Specific Gravity: 1.028

Semen pH: 7.35 to 7.50

Reaction: Alkaline

Chief constituents of seminal fluid:

1. **Fructose:**
   - It is an index of testicular activity.
   - Malnutrition, vitamin deficiency and high fat diet decreases fructose.
   - For ejaculated sperms, fructose is the principal source of energy.
   - Seminal vesicles are chief site of fructose formation.
   - Presence of fructose in semen indicates the patent seminal vesicles.
2. **Sorbitol**
   - Sorbitol, also known as glucitol, is a sugar alcohol, which very slowly metabolises in the body. It is a natural production of the body, but it is poorly digested by the body.
3. **Spermine**
   - Spermine is secreted by the prostate gland, with rich nitrogenous base. The Barberio test, in forensic medicine bears strong diagnostic value when spermine reacts with Picric acid.
   - The crystal of spermine phosphate appears when semen is exposed to room temperature.

4. **Citrate** (Citric Acid)
   - Citrate is derived from the prostatic secretion. Its probable role is to help or enhance the sperm motility.
   - It helps in semen coagulation and liquefaction, because of citric acid having a calcium binding capacity.
   - It helps in activation of prostatic acid phosphatase.
   - It helps in promoting hyaluronidase action.
   - It helps in maintain the osmotic equilibrium in semen

5. **Phosphatase**
   - Acid phosphatase is normally found in male urine in large amount due to admixtures of prostatic secretion.
   - Action of acid phosphatase allows phosphatic acid to accumulate after ejaculation. After then, it reacts with spermine to form spermine phosphate.

6. **Lipids**
   - Lipids in semen are chiefly phospholipids and cholesterol, derived from prostatic secretion. Lipid globules are responsible for the opalescence of the semen. Lipid globules contain macrophages, lipid granules and corpora amylacea, all are from prostate.

7. **Protein: fibrinolysin**
   - Seminal plasma contains 3.5 to 5.5 gm of protein like substance per 100 ml. This 'protein-like substance', perhaps fibrinolysin, is responsible for the coagulation of semen.

8. Choline

- Choline has a nitrogenous base and is always found in high concentration in the human semen.
- It is responsible for physiological functions like –
    - Lipotrophic Activity
    - Stimulation of Phospholipids turn over
    - Transmethylation
    - Acetyl Choline like activity

Choline is crucial for phospholipids metabolism in male accessory organs and for sperms and sperm motility.

9. Ergothioneine

- Like choline, ergothioneine also has a nitrogenous base. It acts as a protective substance for sperm and sperm motility against "sulphydryl group- binding substance" and agents. It acts by preventing oxidation of sulphydryl groups, by ensuring fructose utilisation in sperm and enhancing its motility.

10. Hyaluronidase.

- It derives from the tubule area of the testes, found in semen with the release of the sperm. It is a mucolytic enzyme.
- It depolymerises and hydrolyses the hyaluronic acid. It helps and involves in a process of Spermatogenesis. It facilitates the fertilisation by liquefying passage for each sperm through cumulus cells surrounds the ovum.

11. Prostaglandin

- Prostaglandin is one of a number of hormone-like substances that participate in a wide range of body functions such as the contraction and relaxation of smooth muscle, the dilation and constriction of blood vessels, control of blood pressure and modulation of inflammation. Prostaglandins are derived from a chemical called arachidonic acid.

12. Other substances

The presence of other substances (as mentioned below) in the seminal fluid is also important.

- o Creatine
- o Creatinine
- o Epinephrine
- o Nor-epinephrine
- o Inositol

Outlined above is the basic anatomy and physiology of the male reproductive system, understanding of which is important to justify the clinical condition of the patient.

SPERM:

"Sperm is a male reproductive cell, which unites with the ovum in sexual reproduction to produce a new individual."

The sperm is the end product and outcome of a process known as spermatogenesis, which occurs within the testes. The sperm is a highly motile and polarized cell, which delivers the paternal DNA to the egg or follicle, after conception. The mature sperm is 0.05 millilitres long and consists of a head, body and tail. The head is covered by the crown or cap and contains a nucleus of dense genetic material which contains the 23 chromosomes.

Mature sperm are unable to synthesize nucleic acids and proteins.

Spermatogenesis

- Requires 72 to 74 days for germ-cell maturation i.e. Spermatogonia to mature into spermatozoa
- Most efficient genesis at 34^0 centigrade (93.2^0 Fahrenheit)
- Within the seminiferous tubules, cells of sertolli sustain and regulate the sperm maturation.
- Leydig's cells produce Testosterone.

Basics of Female Reproductive System

It is vital to understand the basic anatomy and physiology of female reproductive system, which comprises of

- Uterus
- Fallopian Tubes
- Ovaries and
- Vagina

Female accessory sex organs like vagina, uterus and fallopian tube (as shown in *Figure 2*) develop from Mulleriano duct.

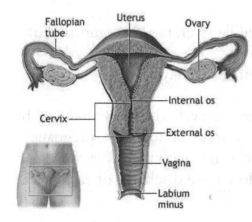

Figure 2 shows the female reproductive system

(http://nursingcrib.com/functions-of-the-female-

OVARIES

Ovaries are pinkish white, ovoid, female reproductive organs. These are homologous to testes in males. They play a prime role in formation of oocytes and production of female sex hormones (like Oestrogen and Progesterone)

Size: 3cm x 1.5cm x 1cm

Shape: Ovoid

Blood Supply: From Ovarian artery which emerges from Aorta, below renal artery.

Venous Drainage: From Pampiniform plexus.
Right Vein drains to Inferior vena cava.
Left Vein drains to Left Renal Vein
Lymph drainage: Lumbar Lymph nodes
Nerve supply: Vaso-motor

UTERUS

Uterus is a thick walled muscular organ, which is the site of foetal development during gestation. It is consists of three layers –

1. Perimetrium (Outermost layer, loose surrounding tissue)
2. Myometrium (Middle layer, mostly comprised of smooth muscle)
3. Endometrium (Innermost layer)

The endometrium undergoes cyclical changes induced by ovarian hormones at the onset of puberty. If, pregnancy does not occur, each cycle ends with menstrual flow produced by the breakdown and discharge of each layer.

Size:
- Length: 7 to 8 cm, Width: 5 cm,
- Thickness: 2.5 cm Weight: 30 to 40 gm.

Shape: Piriform in shape

It is divided in to two parts:
1. The Body - Upper expanded part forms upper 2/3
2. The Cervix - Lower cylindrical part forms lower 1/

The body of the Uterus comprises of
- Fundus
- Two surfaces
- o Anterior or Vesical (towards Urinary bladder)
- o Posterior or Intestinal
- Two Lateral Borders.

The cavity of the uterus is a triangular slit between the intestinal and vesical walls. The uterine tubes enter the angles in the fundus. The apex is continuous with the cervical canal - the junction called the "internal os.

CERVIX

The cervix is cylindrical in shape and is about 2.5 cm long. The canal of cervix is spindle shaped and communicates above with the body of uterus
Blood Supply:
- Arterial Supply:
  1. Chiefly by two Uterine Arteries
  2. Partly by the Ovarian Arteries.
- Lymph drainage:
  - oAortic Nodes
  - oSuperficial Inguinal Nodes
  - oExternal Iliac Nodes
  - oInternal Iliac Nodes
  - oSacral Nodes
- Nerve supply: Inferior Hypogastric Nerve

Important:
- Sympathetic nerves T12 and L1 produce uterine contractions and vaso-constrictions.
- Para-sympathetic nerves S2-S3-S4, produces uterine inhibition and vaso-dilatation.

FALLOPIAN TUBES

Fallopian tubes (also known as oviducts) are lined by ciliated epithelium; and lead from ovaries to uterus. Fallopian Tubes are 10 cm long, muscular structure lined with mucus membrane. The main functions of the Fallopian tube include -

- Transportation of Discharged of ovum
- Fertilisation of ovum

Fallopian tube can be sub-divided into 3 parts -

- Infundibulum: It is the lateral end, Funnel Shaped which contains Fimbria.
- Ampulla: It is the medial to the infundibulum which comprises 6-7 cm of the tube on lateral two-third part of the tube.
- Isthmus: It is 2-3 cm long and comprises medial one third of the tube.

Blood Supply:

- Uterine Artery: to medial two third of the tube
- Ovarian Artery: to lateral one third of the tube.

Venous Drainage:

- Pampiniform Plexus of the ovary and uterine veins.

Lymph Drainage:

- Lateral Aortic Nodes.
- Pre-Aortic Nodes
- Superficial Inguinal Nodes

Nerve Supply:

- Sympathetic Nerves: (T10 to L2) derived from the Hypogastric Plexus.
- Para-sympathetic nerves: derived from the Vagus

VAGINA

Vagina, meaning "sheath" in Latin, is an elastic muscular canal that extends from the cervix to the vulva. It is a female copulatory organ having a fibro muscular tubular tract leading from the cervix of the uterus to the exterior vulva. Although there is wide anatomical variation, the length of the un-aroused vagina is approximately 6 to 7.5 cm (2.5 to 3 in) across the anterior wall (front) and 9 cm (3.5 in) long across the posterior wall (rear). During sexual arousal the vagina expands in both length and width. Its elasticity allows it to stretch during sexual intercourse and during birth to offspring. The vagina connects the superficial vulva to the cervix of the deep uterus.

Structure:

It comprises of four layers.

- Outer most fibrous Layer
- Muscle Layer
- Sub mucus Layer
- Mucus Membrane.

Function of Vagina:

- Excretory canal for menstrual discharge
- Sexual stimulation and orgasmic response during coition
- Receptive for semen pool
- Secretion of various enzymes helps in liquefaction of semen and capacitation of sperms
- Absorbs the seminal prostaglandins
- Acts as birth canal
- Embryological: Female accessory sex organs such as vagina, uterus and fallopian tube develop from Mullerian duct.

Understanding *"physiology of menstruation"*

MENSTRUATION

Shedding of the endometrium (i.e. the uterine lining) is known as menstruation. It is a monthly phenomenon in mammalian females of reproductive age. This phenomenon can also be referred to as the weeping of the uterus for the loss of ovum or the funeral of the unfertilised egg
Regular menstruation (26 to 34 days) always accompanied by Pre - Menstrual Molimina, i.e.

- Breast tenderness
- Lower abdomen bloating
- Moodiness
- All are usually ovulatory.(related to ovulation)

Menstrual cycle – Physiology

Cyclic discharge of blood, mucus and certain other substances from the uterus in the reproductive life of a female, at an average interval of 28 days (24 – 32 days) is called Menstruation.

- It occurs every month from Puberty to Menopause.
- Absence: Before Puberty/ During Pregnancy/After Menopause
- Duration: 4 to 6 days
- Composition:
    o Blood (30 – 50 ml)
    o Stripped of Endometrium
    o Mucus
    o Leucocytes
    o An unfertilised ovum

Four phases of endometrial changes

1. Post Menstrual Phase (Resting phase)
2. Oestrogenic phase (Proliferative phase)
3. Progestetional/Luteal/Pre-Menstrual Phase (Secretary Phase)
4. Menstrual Phase

Phase	Ovarian Changes	Cause
Resting phase Follicular 1 – 5 days	• Degenerated corpus luteum • Action of progesterone: absent • Slowly maturing follicle • ↑ Oestrogen secretion	• Proliferative changes due to oestrogen from the maturing follicle • Controlled by the FSH – Anterior Pituitary
Proliferative phase 6 – 14 days	• Graffian follicle – maturing • Oestrogen secretion - ↑ • On day 14 – ovulation occurs • Corpus luteum formation begins	• Action of oestrogen continuing • Action of FSH is inhibited by ↑ oestrogen level

Luetal phase *Secretory*	• *Growing corpus luteum* • *Secreted progesterone inhibits the further maturation of follicle*	• Due to progesterone • Formation of Corpus luteum and secretion of progesterone are controlled by LH and LTH (Ant Pituitary)
Menstrual phase Starts on 28th day 4 – 6 days Blood Mucus Endometrium Unfertilised ovum	• Degradation of corpus luteum (Placental gonadotrophin is important for further growth of corpus luteum, hence in absence of pregnancy, no placental gonadotrophin present)	

1. ABSINTHIUM

Absinthium=Worm wood always valued as a versatile medicinal plant since1600BC.
Egyptian used it as an "Anti-septic, Stimulant and Tonic.
In Greece, it was used for Rheumatism, Anaemia, Menstrual Colic and easing childbirth

Female:
- Darting Pain in Right Ovary
- Oophoritis
- Ovaralgia
- Atrophy of the ovaries
- Premature Menopause

Male:
- Sexual Neurasthenia
- Spermatorrhoea with relaxed, enfeeble parts

Concomitant:
- Perfect form of epileptic seizures.
- Nervous Tremors followed by an attack of epilepsy.
- Tremors++
- Nervousness++
- Excitement ++

Useful in:

Male:
- Premature Ejaculations

Female:
- Early Menopause
- Peri Menopause
- Right sided Oophoritis.

2. ACETIC ACID

Glacial Acetic Acid: It is produced and excreted by Acetobacter and Clostradium acetobutylicum.In Human, acetic acid is a component of vaginal lubrication serves as an Anti-Bacterial Agent.

Female:

- Excessive Catamania (Profuse Menstruation)
      (Kata= monthly, moon, menses means Heavy
      periods-DUB, Metrorrhagia)
- Nausea after pregnancy
- Breasts painfully enlarged, distended with milk.
- Milk= impoverished, Bluish, Transparent, Sour.
- Haemorrhage after labour.
- Anaemia of nursing mother.
- <u>Mind:</u> Irritable, worried about business affairs.

Concomitant:

- Anaemia, Dropsy, Great debility, Frequent Fainting,
- Dyspnoea, wasting and debility.

Note:
1. Acetic acid has the power to liquefy albuminous and fibrinous deposits.
2. Epithelial Cancer –internally and locally.
3. Sycosis with nodules and nodules formation in the joints.

Useful in:

- DUB=Dysfunctional Uterine Bleeding
- PPH= Postpartal Haemorrhage
- Hyperemesis Gravidarum
- PCM=Protein Caloric Malnutrition
- Anaemia
- Thyroid dysfunction
- Mastitis
- Cancer
- Osteoporosis with Formation of osteophytes in Joints

3. ACONITE NAPALLUS

Monkshood well described in Greek and Romans as Anodyne, Diuretic and Diaphoretic. Acts on circulation, respiration and nervous system.

Male:
- Crawling and stinging in the Glans
- Bruised pain in the testicles
- Testicles: Swollen, Hard
- Frequent emissions and Erections
- Painful erection

Female:
- Vagina: Dry, Hot Sensitive
- Uterus: Sharp, Shooting pains in the womb
- Ovaries: Congested and Painful
- Frenzy on appearance of Menses.
- Fear and Restlessness after pain.
- Menses:
    - Too profuse with Epistaxis,
    - Too protracted
    - Late

Concomitant:
- Physical and Mental Restlessness

Useful in:
Male:
- Orchitis
- Premature Ejaculations

Female:
- Vaginal Dryness
- Oophoritis

4. AESCULUS HIPPOCASTANUM

(Hoarse chestnut)
Its extract is widely used for chronic venous insufficiency=CVI, presenting Leg swelling, varicose veins, Leg pains, Itching and Skin Ulcers.

Male:

- Discharge of prostatic fluid at stool

Female:

- Constant throbbing behind Symphysis Pubis
- Leucorrhoea: Dark, Yellow, Sticky, Corroding
  Worst: after menses

Concomitant:

- Lameness of back across the Sacro-Iliac articulation.

Note:
The saponin aescin (a complex mixture of triterpene glycosides), however, has been used for health purposes (such as varicose veins, edema, sprains) and is available in food supplements, as is the coumarin glucoside.

5. AETHUSA CYNAPIUM
(Fool's parsley)

Female:

- Lancinating pains in sexual organs.
- Pimples: on face
- Itching when warm on Cheeks.
- Menses: Watery
- Breast:
  Swelling of Mammary gland with lancinating pain.

Useful in:

- Mastitis
- Thrush-Moniliasis, Candida etc.

6. AGARICUS MUSCARIUS AMANITA

Toad stool - Bug Agaric-Amanita Muscaria was widely used in Siberia as an Entheogen having psychoactive property and was used for recreational purpose like Hallucinogen-producing effects such as euphoria, relaxation, changes in mood.

Male:

- Aspermia
- Sexual desire increased in morning on waking.
- Hysteria after sex.
- Fainting.

Female:

- Menses: Increased earlier
- Itching and tearing pain
- Pressive pain of Genitalia and Back
- Spasmodic Dysmenorrhoea
- Severe bearing down pain esp. after menopause
- Sexual Excitement
- Nipples: Itch, Burn
- Complains following parturition and coition
- Leucorrhoea with much itching.

Useful in:

Male

- Aspermia
- Hysteria after sex

Female

- Spasmodic Dysmenorrhoea
- Excoriation of Nipples
- Leucorrhoea with Itching

7. AGNUS CASTUS

Chaste tree-Originally used as Anti-Libido Medicine by monks to maintain chastity, as anaphrodisiac. It's having a Dopaminergic effect, affecting prolactin secretion by inhibiting activation of dopamine2 receptor. Any reduction in prolactin influences FSH and Oestrogen secretion in females and Testosterone in men.

Male:
- Yellow discharge from Urethra.
- Impotence
- Parts Cold, Relaxed
- Desire gone. (Conium, Sabal, Selenium)
- Scanty emission without ejaculation.
- Loss of prostatic fluid on straining.
- Gleety Discharge
- Testicles: Cold, Swollen, Hard, Painful

Female:
- Sterility
- Abhorrence(Fear, Loathe) of Sexual Intercourse
- Relaxation of Genitalia with Leucorrhoea
- Leucorrhoea : Staining Yellow, Transparent
- Menses: Scanty

Concomitant:
- Hysterical Palpitation with Epistaxis
- Breasts: Agalactia with sadness

Useful in:
Male:
- Impotence
- Erectile dysfunction

Female:
- Sterility
- Agalactia

8. ALETRIS FARINOSA

Star grass-Known as a white colic root, was used as an Emetic, Narcotic, Cathartic and Uterine tonic with Anti-abortive and female restorative properties.

Female:

- Anaemic
- Tired and Relax -all the time suffers from
    o Prolapsus Uteri
    o Leucorrhoea
    o Rectal Distress
- Menses:
    o Premature and Profuse with labour like pain
    o Retarded and Scanty flow
- Uterus: Heavy
- Uterine prolapse with pain in Right Inguinal Fossa
- Leucorrhoea due to weakness and Anaemia
- Tendency to Habitual Abortion
- Muscular pain during pregnancy

Useful in:

Female:

- Anaemia related Leucorrhoea
- Tendency to abort-Habitual Abortion
- Endometriosis
- Prolapse of Uterus.
- Bacterial Vaginitis
- Oligo-menorrhoea
- Cervical Erosion
- Incompetent Os.

9. ALFA ALFA
(Medicago Sativa)

Medicago Sativa is an Immuno booster, rich in calcium, minerals, and Vitamin-B group, Vitamin-C, Vitamin-E and Vitamin-K.
Useful in Arthritis and water retention.

Male:

- In benign Hyperplasia of prostate.
- It relieves Vesical Irritability=Irritable Bladder.
- Good for Senile Irritable Bladder.

Female:
- Deficient Lactation
- Increases quality and quantity of milk in nursing mothers.
- Galactogogue.

Useful in:

Male:
- Sexual Neurasthenia
- Toning-up
- Improves mental and physical vigour

Female:
- Corrects tissue waste
- Improves Lactation
- Improves the quality of Milk in Nursing Mothers

10. ALLIUM SATIVUM

Garlic is Anti-bacterial, Anti-fungal and Anti-viral and Anti-helminthic properties. It contains *Allicin* which is powerful Anti-biotic and *Phytoncide,* which considered having Anti-oxidative, Anti-microbial and Anti-tumour properties. It enhances Thiamine absorption and prevents Beri-Beri. It helps to regulate the blood sugar.

Female:

- Pain and swelling of Breasts.
- Eruptions in Vagina, on breasts & vulva during menses.
- Suitable to meat eaters.

Useful in:

Female:

- Improves the Intestinal flora and corrects the chronic Fungal Infections like Thrush.
- Expels out the Chronic Worm infestation
- Great Anti-septic

11. ALNUS RUBRA

Red Alder was being used to treat poison oak, insect bites and skin irritation. It contains *Betulin* and *Lupeol*-both are effective against variety of tumours.

Female:

- Leucorrhoea with cervical erosion, Cervix becomes Red, Spongy
- Bleeding on touch – Bleeds easily on gynaecological examinations.
- Amenorrhoea with burning pains from back to pubis.

Useful in:

Female:

- Relieves any type of mucosal Irritation
- Cervical Erosion
- Cervix –Red, Spongy
- It helps in preventing bleeding.

12. ALOE
(Socotrine Aloe)

Socotrine Aloe is an Immuno-stimulant with Anti-bacterial and Anti-Fungal properties which inhibits the growth of Tinea.

Male:
- Impotency

Female:

- Bearing down in rectum
- All Complains aggravated from standing and during menses
- Uterus: Feels Heavy, Can not walk much on that account.
- Labour like pains in loins, extended down legs.
- Climacteric Haemorrhages
- Menses: Too early and too profuse.

Useful in:

Male:
- Impotency

Female:

- Uterine Hyperplasia with Intestinal Irritation
- Endometriosis (Dyschasia)
- Menopausal Bleeding

13. ALUMEN

Common Potash Alum is being used as an Astringent, Anti-bacterial and Deodorant. Widely used as an Immunological adjuvant (means any substance that acts to accelerate, prolong or enhance Antigen Specific Immune Response when used with vaccine) It is also used as an ingredient in loose vaginal tightening cream.

Female:

- Tendency to indurations of neck of Uterus
- Induration of Mammary Glands
- Leucorrhoea
- Chronic Yellow Vaginal Discharge
- Chronic Gonorrhoea-Yellow with little lump along urethra
- Apthous patches in Vagina
- Menses; Watery

Useful in:

Female:

- Chronic Vaginal Discharge-Leucorrhoea
- Leads to indurations of neck of uterus
- Leads to Cervical Stenosis
- Chronic Vaginitis
- Fibro adenoma of Breasts.

14. ALUMINA
(Argilla-Oxide of Aluminium)

Male:
- Excessive desire
- Prostatic Discharge
- Involuntary emission at straining at stool

Female:
- Hasty, hurried with variable mood
- Menses: Too early, Short, Scanty, Pale…followed by
- Great Exhaustion
- Leucorrhoea: Acrid, Profuse, Transparent, and Ropy with Burning.
- Better: after Washing with Cold Water

Useful in:

Male:
- Increased Desire
- Involuntary Emissions

Female:
- Leucorrhoea: Acrid

15. AMBRA GRISEA
(Ambergis - A morbid Secretion of Whale)

Biliary secretion of the intestine of the sperm whale, used as flavouring agent and as an Aphrodisiac. During the middle Ages, Europeans used ambergris as a medication for headaches, colds, epilepsy, and other ailments.

Male:

- Voluptuous itching of Scrotum
- Parts extremely numb
- Violent Erections without voluptuous sensations.

Female:

- Itching of pudendum with soreness and Swelling
- Discharge of blood between periods, at every little accident.
- Menses: Too early, Too profuse.
- Leucorrhoea: Bluish- Worse: at night
- Extreme Nervous Hypersensitiveness
- Nymphomania

Useful in:

Male:

- Itching of Scrotum
- Violent Erections

Female:

- Itching of Pudenda
- Nymphomania

16. AMMONIUM CARB.

Male:

- Pain, Inflammation and Itching of Scrotum and Spermatic Cords.
- Erections without desire.
- Seminal Emissions

Female:

- Stout women-always tired and weary.
- Catches Cold easily,
- Usually leads a sedentary life with always Slow Reaction
- Itching, Swelling and burning of pudendum.
- Leucorrhoea: Burning, Acrid, Watery
- Aversion to the opposite sex.
- Cholera Like symptoms before menses.
- Menses: Too frequent, Early, Profuse, Copious, Clotted and Black.
- Colicky pain and hard difficult stool with fatigue of thighs.
- Yawning and Chilliness.

Useful in:

Male:

- Scrotal Pruritus
- Decreased Libido

Female

- Catches Cold easily
- Frigidity
- DUB (Dysfunctional Uterine Bleeding)

17. AMMONIUM MURIATICUM
(Sal Ammoniac)

Male:

- Lack of emotional warmth and no erection.
- Do not express feeling during act. No interest.
- Always feels tired and sore, so avoiding act.
- Deeply affected grief made him withdrawn.

Female:

- Menses:
- Too early, too free, too dark, clotted.
- Flow more at night.
- During Pregnancy: Pain in Left Iliac Fossa, as if, sprained.
- During menses:
- Diarrhoea: Greenish mucus mixed stool and Pain around Umbilical Region.
- Leucorrhoea:
- Like: White of an Egg with pain around Umbilicus.
- After every Urination: Leucorrhoea brown and Slimy.

Useful in:

Male:

- Deeply affected Grief
- No expression of feelings
- Always tired
- No desire

Female:

- DUB
- Pain in LIF during Pregnancy
- Leucorrhoea like white of an egg
- Candidasis-Moniliasis

18. AMYGDALUS PERSICA
(Peach Tree)

Female:
- Morning Sickness
- Constant Nausea and Vomiting
- Hyper emesis Gravidarum
- Haemorrhage from Bladder.

Useful in:

Female:
- Hyper emesis Gravidarum
- Haematuria

19. AMYL NITROSUM
(Amyl Nitrate)

Female:
- After-Pains
- Haemorrhage associated with Facial Flushing
- Climacteric Headache
- Flushes of Heat with anxiety and Palpitation
- All complains gets aggravated at menopause.

Useful in:
Female:
- Menopausal Headache
- Menopausal Anxiety
- Frequent Hot flushes

20. ANACARDIUM
(Marking Nut)

Male:
- Voluptuous Itching
- Increased Desire
- Seminal Emissions without Dreams
- Prostatic Discharge during stool

Female:
- Menses: Scanty
- Leucorrhoea: with soreness and Itching

Useful in:

Male:
- Pruritus
- Increased Sexual Desire
- Nocturnal Seminal emissions

Female:

- Leucorrhoea associated with pruritus

21. ANATHERUM

(Cuscus - an East Indian Grass)

Female:
Sexual Symptoms:
- Chancre – like sores.
- Scirrhus-like Swelling of Cervix.
- Breast: Swollen, Indurate
- Nipples: Excoriated.

Useful in:

Female:
- Tendency to form Ulcers
- Cervical Erosion-Swelling
- Breast Swelling
- Fibro adenoma of Breast
- Nipples are cracked

22. ANTHRACINUM
(Anthrax poison)

In Greek, Anthrax means Anthracite means coal, which refers to – intolerable burning and that is the chief Characteristic of disease.

- Haemorrhages: Black, Thick, Tar-Like
- Rapidly decomposing from any orifice.
- Glands: Swollen, Inflamed, Indurate
- Septicaemia
- Gangrene
- Ulceration with Intolerable Burning.

23. ANTIMONIUM CRUDUM
(Black Sulphide of Antimony)

Male:
- Eruptions on scrotum and around Genitals.
- Impotence
- Atrophy of Penis and Testes.

Female:
- Itching on parts makes her excited
- Toothache before menses
- Menses: Too Early, Too Profuse
- Menses: Suppressed from Cold Bathing.
- With feeling of Pressure in pelvis
- Tenderness in ovarian region.
- Leucorrhoea: Watery, Acrid, Lumpy

Useful in:

Male:
- Impotence
- Atrophy of penis
- Atrophy of Testes
- Scrotal Eruptions

Female:

- Suppressed Menses
- Oophoritis (ovary inflammation)
- Salpingitis(Inflammation of fallopian tube)

24. ANTIMONIUM IODATUM

Female:

- Uterine Hyperplasia
- Endometriosis

25. ANTIPYRINE

(Phenazone- a coal tar derivative)

Female:

- Itching and Burning in Vagina.
- Menses: Suppressed
- Watery Leucorrhoea

26. APIS MELLIFICA
(Honey Bee)

Female:

- Oedema of Labia-Relieved by Cold water.
- Soreness and Stinging Pain
- Ovaritis esp. Worse in RIGHT OVARY.
- Menses Suppressed with Cerebral and Head Symptoms, esp. in Young Girls.
- Dysmenorrhoea: with severe Ovarian Pain.
- Metrorrhagia: Profuse Bleeding with heavy abdomen, faintness and stinging pains.
- Sense of tightness.
- Bearing down sensation-as if menses were to appear.
- Ovarian tumours.
- Metritis (inflammation of the womb) with stinging pain.
- Great tenderness over abdomen and uterine region.

HOW APIS WORKS?

The sting of bee, wasp, Fire ants and insects contains...
1. Phospholipase A2
2. Hyaluronidase
3. Apamin
4. Melitin
5. Kinins.

PATHO-PHYSIOLOGY OF BEE STING

- After bee sting...
- Body quickly over reacts with Histamine secretion
- Bee Sting triggers up the release of Histamine from Mast Cells.
- Histamine is usually found in higher concentration in Skin, Lungs and in Gastric Mucosa.
- Histamine is a potent arterial dilator leading to Hypotension.
- Histamine is a potent arterial dilator leading to Hypotension.
- In lungs, it causes Bronchial constriction leading to spasm, dyspnoea, wheezing and Respiratory collapse.

Phospholipase A2...

Its membrane Protein, which hydrolyzes

↓

Phospholipids...to form...

↓

Fatty Acids and Lysophosholipid products.

↓

Phospholipase A2 proteins are responsible for the release of...

Archidonic Acid from Cell Membrane.

- Subsequent conversion of this Fatty Acid to ...
- Leukotrienes and Prostaglandin is a part of inflammatory response.
- Leading to Inflammatory cyst formation.
- APIS MELLIFICA is working to remove the cysts from the ovaries.

27. APIUM GRAVEOLENS
(Common Celery)

Female:

- Sharp, sticking pain in both OVARIAN Regions.
- Better by: Left side.
- Lying on and bending with flexed legs.
- Nipples: Tender.

28. APOCYNUM CANNABINUM
(Indian hemp)

Female:

- Amenorrhoea with Bloating
- Metrorrhagia with Nausea and Fainting.
- Vital Depression
- Haemorrhages at Change of Life. (Menopausal)
- Blood expelled in large clots.

29. AQUILEGIA
(Columbine)

Female:

- Globus Hystericus
- Clayus Hystericus
- Women at Climaxes
- Dysmenorrhoea of Young Girls.
- Menses: Scanty, Dull, Painful,
- Nightly, increasing pressure in Right Lumbar Region.

30. ARALIA RACEMOSA
(American Spikenard)

Female:

- Menses: Suppressed.
- Leucorrhoea: Foul Smelling, Acrid with pressing down pain.
- Lochia: Suppressed with Tympanitis

31. ARANEA DIADEMA
(Papal cross spider)

Female:

- Menses: Too Early, Too Copious
- Dissention of Abdomen
- Lumbo-abdominal Neuralgia.

32. ARGEMONE MAXICANA
(Prickly Poppy)

Female:

- Menses: Suppressed.
- Diminished Sexual Desire with Weakness.

33. ARGENTUM METTALICUM.
(Silver-the Metal)

Male:

- Testicles: Crushed Pain
- Seminal Emissions without excitement.
- Frequent Micturition with Burning.

Female:

- Ovaries: Feels too large.
- Pain in Left Ovary.
- Bearing down pain.
- Prolapsed of Uterus.
- Cervical Erosion-Eroded Spongy Cervix.
- Leucorrhoea: Foul, Excoriating.
- Palliative in scirrhus of uterus.
  (A hard dense cancerous growth usually arising from connective tissue)
- Climacteric Haemorrhages.
- Uterine Diseases with pain in Joints and Limbs.
- Sore Feeling through out abdomen.
- Worse by Jarring.

34. ARGENTUM NITRICUM
(Nitrite of Silver)

Male:
- Impotence
- Erection fails when coition attempted
- Desire wanting
- Genitals Shrivel.
- Coition Painful.
- Cancer like Ulcers.

Female:
- Gastralgia at the beginning of menses.
- Intense spasm of Chest Muscles.
- Orgasms at Night
- Nervous Erethism at change of life (Menopause)
- Leucorrhoea: Profuse with Cervical Erosion.
- Bleeds easily.
- Uterine Haemorrhage - Two weeks after menses.
- Painful affection of LEFT Ovary.

Important Facts about Argentum Nitricum- SILVER

- Hippocrates wrote: SILVER had beneficial healing and anti-disease property.
- During ancient civilisation: SILVER used to store water, wine, vinegar-to prevent spoiling.
- During 1900, people used to put silver Dollars in milk bottle to preserve the freshness of milk.
- During world war-1, silver compound widely and successfully used to prevent infection.

- Some Indian sweets, silver foil used as a preservative.
- In Dentistry, silver filling in tooth widely used to prevent decay.
- Silver possesses property to treat Burns and Pain Reduction.
- Alginate, SEA WEEDS, kelp, Macrocystis Pyrifera for Burns and wound Victims which contains Silver. Alginate used in Gaviscone and in Bisodol.
- Samsung has introduced Washing Machine which contains SILVER IONS to finish Final Rinse to provide Anti-Bacterial Protection.
- FDA-USA approved Endo-tracheal tube, for mechanical Ventilation with a coat of SILVER---to reduce the risk of VENTILATOR associated Pnuemonia-ASPIRATION Pneumonia.
- SILVER widely used in Religious celebration everywhere.

With all these, we can conclude, Silver having ...

- Anti-Inflammatory property
- Anti-septic property
- Anti-Bacterial Property
- Preservative and Restorative Property
- Anti-Fungal and Healing Agent.

So, Argentum Nitricum removes inflammatory reactions to testes & restores Deranged Pathology back to normal enhancing the normal Spermatogenesis, making to improve his pre-conceptional problem of Oligo-spermia to Normal Sperm count.

35. ARNICA.

(Leopard's Bane)

Male:

- Benign Hyperplasia of Prostate ,hence Ribbon Like stools.

Female:

- Bruised parts after Labour.
- Violent after-Pains.
- Uterine Haemorrhage from mechanical Injury after coition.
- Mastitis: Sore Nipples-from Injury.
- Feeling-as if Foetus were lying Cross-wise.

36. ARSENICUM ALBUM
(Arsenious Acid - Arsenic Trioxide)
Female:

- Menses: Too profuse and Too soon-early.
- Burning in Ovarian Region.
- Leucorrhoea: Acrid, Burning, Offensive, and Thin.
- Pain as from Red-Hot Wires, Worse from least exertion. Causes great fatigue-Better in Warm Room.
- Menorrhagia:
- Stitching Pain in pelvis extending down the thighs.

37. ARTEMISIA VULGARIS
(Mug wort)

Female:
- Profuse Menses.
- Violent Uterine Contractions
- Spasm during menses.

38. ARUNDO
(Reed)

Male:

- Pain in Spermatic Cord after Embrace.

Female:

- Menses: Too early-Too profuse.
- Neuralgic pain from Face to Shoulders and Pubis.
- Desire with Vaginal Pruritus.
- Burning and Pain in Nipples.

39. ASAFOETIDA
(Gum of the stink sand)

Female:

- Mammae Turgid with Milk in the Unimpregnated.
- Deficient Milk with over sensitiveness.

40. ASARUM EUROPEUM
(European Snake –Root)

Female:

- Menses: Too early, Long Lasting, Black.
- Violent pain in small of back.
- Leucorrhoea: Tenacious, Yellow.

41. ASTERIAS RUBENS

(Red Star Fish)

Female:

- Colic and other sufferings ceases with appearance of flow.
- Breast: Swell, Pain in Breast-Worse on Left.
- Ulceration with sharp pains, piercing to Scapulae.
- Pains down the Left arm to the Fingers.
- Worse: by Motion.
- Excitement with Sexual Instinct with Nervous Agitation.
- Breasts: Nodules and Inflammatory Changes. Induration of mammary glands.
- Dull, Aching, Neuralgic Pain in Pectoral Region.

42. AURUM METALLICUM
(Gold-the metal)

Male:

Every opportunity is sought for Self-Destruction.
- Pain and Swelling of Testicles.
- Chronic Indurations of Testes.
- Violent Erections.
- Atrophy of Testicles in Boys.
- Hydrocele.

Female:

- Great Sensitiveness of Vagina.
- Uterus enlarged and prolapsed.
- Sterility.
- Vaginismus.

43. AURUM MURIATICUM NATRONATUM
(Sodium Chloroaurate)

Female:

- Indurated Cervix.
- Palpitation of Young Girls.
- Coldness in abdomen.
- Chronic Metritis and Prolapsus.
- Uterus fills up whole pelvis- Enlargement.
- Ulceration of neck of Uterus- Isthmus and Vagina.
- Ovaries: indurated.
- Ovarian dropsy.
- Sub involution.
- Ossified uterus.

44. AVENA SATIVA
(Common Oat)

Male:

- Spermatorrhoea
- Impotency- after too much indulgence.

Female:

- Amenorrhoea
- Dysmenorrhoea with weak circulation.

45. BADIAGA
(Fresh Water Sponge)

Female:

- Metrorrhagia: Worse at Night with feeling of
- Enlargement of Head.
- Cancer of Breast.

46. BAPTISIA.
(Wild Indigo)

Male:
- Testicular Atrophy

Female:
- Threatened Abortion.
- Miscarriage from Mental Depression, Shock,
- Low fever.
- Menses: Too Early, Too Profuse.
- Lochia: Acrid, Foetid.
- Puerperal Fever.

Useful in:

Male
- Testicular Atrophy.

Female
- Threatened Abortion
- Puerperal Fever

47. BAROSMA CRENATA
(Buchu)

Female:

- Muco-purulent Discharge
- Leucorrhoea
- Irritable Bladder.

Useful in:

Female:
- Irritable Bladder
- Leucorrhoea

48. BARYTA CARB
(Carbonate of Baryta)

Male:
- Diminished Desire.
- Premature Impotence
- Enlarged Prostate
- Induration of Testicles.

Female:
- Pain in stomach and small of back.
- Menses: Scanty
- Prevents: Degenerative Changes.

49. BARYTA MURIATICUM
(Barium Chloride)

Male:

- Satyriasis.
- The sexual desire is always increased, in every form of Mania.

Female:

- Nymphomania.

Useful in:

Male

- Satyriasis(Excessive or abnormal craving for sex)
- Hyper sexuality.

Female:

- Nymphomania

50. BELLADONNA
(Deadly night shed)

Male:

- Testicles: Hard, Drawn up, Inflamed.
- Nocturnal Sweat of Genitals.
- Flow of prostatic Fluid.
- Desire: Diminished.

Female:
- Sensation as if- all the viscera would protrude at genitals.
- Sensitive forcing downward.
- Dryness and Heat of Vagina.
- Dragging around Loins.
- Pain in Sacrum.
- Menses: Increased, Bright red, too early, Too Profuse, Haemorrhages hot.
- Cutting Pain from Hip to Hip.
- Menses and Lochia: Very Offensive and Hot.
- Labour Pains: Comes and Goes Suddenly.
- Breasts: Mastitis: Throbbing pain, Redness, Streaks radiates from Nipple.
- Breasts Feels: Heavy, Hard and Red.
- Tumours of Breasts.
- Pain: Worse Lying down.
- Badly Smelling Haemorrhage.
- Hot gushes of Blood.
- Diminished Lochia.

51. BENZENUM - COAL NAPHTHA
(Benzol)

Male:
- Swelling of Right Testicle.
- Severe Pain in Testicles.
- Itching of Scrotum.
- Profuse Urination.

Useful in:

Male:
- Right Testicular Swelling
- Right Sided Orchitis
- Scrotal Itching

52. BERBERIS VULGARIS.
(Berberry)

Male:

- Neuralgia of Spermatic Cord and Testicles.
- Smarting, Burning, and Stitching in Testicles, esp. in Prepuce and Scrotum.

Female:

- Vaginismus.
- Pinching Constriction in Mons Veneris.
- Contractions and Tenderness of Vagina.
- Burning and Soreness in Vagina.
- Desire: Diminished.
- Cutting Pain during Coition.
- Menses: Scanty, Gray mucus with pain in Kidneys and Chilliness.
- Pain down the thighs.
- Leucorrhoea: Greyish mucus with painful Urinary Symptoms.
- Neuralgia of Ovaries and Vagina.

Useful in:

Male:

- Orchitis

Female:

- Vaginismus
- Frigidity
- Right Oophoritis.

53. BORICUM ACIDUM
(Boracic Acid)

Female:
- Climacteric Flushing.
- Vagina: Cold-as if packed with Ice.
- Urination with Burning and Tenesmus.

Useful in:

Female:
- Menopausal Hot Flushes
- Burning Urination

54. BORAX
(Borate of Sodium)

Female:
- Labour Pains with frequent eructation.
- Galactorhhoea.
- While nursing, pain in opposite Breast.
- Leucorrhoea: Like an egg white with sensation as if Warm water was flowing.
- Menses: Too soon, Profuse with griping pain in stomach and Nausea, extending to small of back.
- Membranous Dysmenorrhoea.
- Sterility
- Favours easy conception.
- Sensation of Distention in Clitoris with sticking.
- Pruritus Vulva associated with Eczema.

Useful in:
Female:
- Excellent medicines for Moniliasis.
- Sterility
- Galactorrhoea
- Favours conception.

55. BOVISTA
(Puff Ball)

Female:
- Diarrhoea: before and during menses.
- Menses: Too early, Too Profuse, Aggravation at night.
- Voluptuous Sensations.
- Leucorrhoea: Acrid, Thick, Tough, Greenish followed by Menses.
- Can not bear tight clothing around waist.
- Traces of menses between menstruations.
- Soreness of pubis during menstruation.
- Para ovarian cysts.

56. BROMIUM
(Bromine)

Male:
- Swelling of Testicles:
- Indurate with Pain.
- Worse: Slightest Jar.

Female:
- Swelling of ovaries.
- Menses: Too Early, Too Profuse with membranous shreds.
- "Low Spirited" before menses.
- Breasts: Tumour in Breasts with stitching pain.
- Worse: Left Breast
- Stitching Pain from Breast to axilla.
- Sharp, shooting pain in Left Breast.
- Worse: by pressure.

Useful in:
Male:
- Orchitis
- Testicular Swelling
- Indurations-Testes
- Tenderness

Female:
- Oophoritis
- Endometriosis
- Tumours in Breast

57. BRYONIA ALBA
(Wild Hops)

Female:

- Menses: Too early, Too profuse.
- Worse: from Motion with tearing pain in legs.
- Menses: Suppressed with Vicarious Discharge or Splitting headache.
- Stitching pain in ovaries on taking a deep breath(Inspiration)
- Very sensitive to touch.
- Pain in Right Ovary-as if torn, extending to thigh.
- Milk fever.
- Pain in breast at menstruation.
- Breasts: Hot, Painful, Hard.
- Abscess of Mammae.
- Frequent bleeding from nose-Epistaxis, at the appearance of menses. Vicarious menstruation.
- Menstrual Irregularities with Gastric Symptoms.
- Ovaritis.
- Inter menstrual pain with great abdominal and pelvic soreness.

58. BUFO RANA
(Poison of Toad)

Male:
- Impotence
- Involuntary emissions
- Discharge: Too Quick.
- Spasms during coition.
- Buboes(An inflamed, tender swelling of lymph node)
- Disposition to handle organ.
- Effects of Onanism. (Manual stimulation of own organ for sexual pleasure)

Female:
- Menses: Too early and Copious.
- Clots and Bloody Discharge at other time.
- Leucorrhoea: Watery.
- Excitement with Epileptic Attacks.
- Epilepsy at the time of Menses.
- Breasts: Indurations of Mammary Glands.
- Proved effective as a Palliative in Breast Cancer.
- Burning in Ovaries and Uterus.
- Ulceration of Cervix.
- Offensive bloody discharge.
- Pain runs in to the legs.
- Bloody milk.
- Milk leg. (Phlegmesia alba dolens)
- Veins: Swollen. (Thrombo-phlebitis)
- Tumours and Polypii of Uterus.

59. CACTUS GRANDIFLORUS.

(Night blooming Cereus)

Female:

- Constriction in Uterine Region and Ovarian Region.
- Dysmenorrhoea.
- Pulsating pain in uterus and ovaries.
- Vaginismus.
- Menses: early, dark, pitch like.
- Ceases on lying down with Heart Symptoms.

60. CAHINCA

(Brazilian Plant - chiococca)

Male:

- Drawing pain of Testicles and Spermatic Cord.
- Pain: Worse: While passing pungent smelling Urine.

61. CALADIUM SEGUINUM
(American Arum)

Male:
- Pruritus.
- Glands very red.
- An organ seems larger, puffed, relaxed, cold, sweating.
- Scrotum: Skin: Very Thick.
- Impotency.
- Erections: When half asleep, ceases when fully awake.
- Relaxation of penis during excitement.
- No Emissions and No Orgasm, during embrace.

Female:
- Pruritus of vulvae and vagina, during pregnancy.
- Voluptuousness.
- Cramping pain in Uterus at night.

62. CALCAREA ACETICA
(Acetate of Lime)

Female:

- Membranous Dysmenorrhoea.
- Membranous Exudation.
- Cancer Pain.

63. CALCAREA ARSENICA
(Arsenate of Lime)

Female:

- Leucorrhoea-Offensive, Bloody.
- Cancer of Uterus.
- Burning Pain in Uterus and Vagina

64. CALCAREA CARBONICA
(Carbonate of Lime)

Male:

- Frequent Emissions
- Increased Desire.
- Semen emitted too soon.(Premature Ejaculations)
- Coition followed by weakness and Irritability.
- Over exhausted state-mental and Physical due to over work- often noticed as-"Jaded state".

Female:

- Before Menses - Pre Menstrual complains like,
- Headache, Colic, Chilliness and Leucorrhoea.
- Cutting Pain in Uterus during menstruation.
- Menses: Too early, Too Profuse, Too long lasting with Vertigo, Toothache and Cold damp feet. The least excitement causes their return.
- Uterus: Easily Displaced.
- Leucorrhoea: Milky.
- Burning and Itching of parts: before menses and after menses - especially in little Girls.
- Increased Sexual Desire.
- Easy conception.
- Breasts: Tender and swollen before menses.
- Milk: Too abundant- Disagreeable to child.
- In Lymphatic Women: Deficient Lactation with Distended Breasts.
- Much sweat around external Genitals.
- Sterility with copious menses.
- Uterine polypii.

65. CALCAREA FLOURICA

(Fluoride of Lime)

Male:

- Powerful tissue remedy for Hard, Stony Glands.
- Enlarged Veins
- Varicose Veins.
- Hydrocele.
- Induration of testes.

Female:

- Powerful tissue remedy for Hard, Stony Glands.
- Hard Knots in Female Breasts.
- If used after any operation, it reduces adhesions and fibrosis.

66. CALCAREA PHOSPHORICA
(Phosphate of Lime)

Female:
- Menses: Too early, Excessive and bright, in School Girls.
- If menses comes late: Then blood is dark, sometime first bright and then dark with violent Backache. (Premenstrual syndrome)
- Sexual Excitement with Lactation.
- Nymphomania with aching, pressing and weakness in uterine region—after prolonged nursing.
- Leucorrhoea: like White of an Egg, Worse: Morning.
- Child refuses breast: milk taste salty.
- Prolapsus in debilitated person.

67. CALCAREA SILICATA
(Silicate of Lime)

Female:
- Suitable to Hydrogenoid Constitution.
- Uterus: Heavy, Prolapsed.
- Leucorrhoea: Painful
- Menses: Irregular.
- Flow between periods

68. CALENDULA OFFICINALIS
(Marigold)

Female:

- Warts: at the External Os of Uterus.
- Menses: Suppressed with Cough.
- Chronic endocervicitis.
- Uterine hypertrophy.
- Sensation of Weight and Fullness in pelvis.
- Stretching and dragging in groin.
- Pain on sudden movement.
- Os lower than natural. ? Elongated Cervix. ? Prolapse
- Menorrhagia.

Useful in:

Female:

- Endocervicitis
- Uterine Hypertrophy
- Endometriosis

69. CAMPHORA
(Camphor)

Male:

- Desire Increased.
- Chordee
- Priapism
- Nightly Emissions
- Icy coldness of parts.

70. CANNABIS INDICA.
(Hashish)

Male:
- Backache after Sexual Intercourse.
- Oozing of white, glary mucus from Glans.
- Satyriasis.
- Prolonged thrill.
- Chordee.
- Sensation of swelling in perineum or Perianal region.
- Sensation- "as if Sitting on a Ball."

Female:

- Menses: Profuse, Dark, Painful without clots.
- Backache during menses.
- Uterine Colic with great nervous agitation associated with sleepiness.
- Sterility
- Dysmenorrhoea with Sexual Desire.

71. CANNABIS SATIVA
(Hemp)

Female:

- Amenorrhoea-When physical power has been over taxed, with Constipation.

72. CANTHARIS
(Spanish fly)

Male:

- Strong Desire with painful erections.
- Pain in Glans.
- Priapism in Gonorrhoea.

Female:

- Retained Placenta with Painful Urination.
- Expels: Moles, Dead Foetus, and Membranes etc.
- Nymphomania
- Puerperal metritis with inflammation of Bladder.
- Menses: Too early and Too profuse.
- Black Swelling of Vulva with irritation.
- Constant Discharge from Uterus.
- Burning Pain in Ovaries, extremely sensitive.
- Lancinating and Tearing Coccygeal Pain.

73. CAPSICUM
(Cayenne pepper)

Male:
- Coldness of Scrotum with Impotency.
- Testicular Atrophy.
- Loss of Sensation in Testicles.
- Testicular Softening and Dwindling.
- Gonorrhoea with Chordee.
- Excessive Burning Pain in Prostate.

Female:
- Climacteric Disturbance with burning of tip of tongue.
- Uterine Haemorrhage near the Menopause associated with nausea
- Sticking sensation in left ovarian region.

74. CARBO ANIMALIS
(Animal Charcoal)

Female:

- Nausea at Pregnancy-Worse at night.
- Lochia-Offensive.
- Menses: Too Early, frequent, long lasting followed by great exhaustion.
- Very Weak, Can hardly speak.
- Menstrual Flow: only in Morning.
- Burning in Vagina and Labia.
- Breasts: Darting in Breast
- Right sided- Painful indurations in Breast.
- Cancer of Uterus.
- Burning pain down thighs.

75. CARBO VEGETABILIS
(Vegetable Charcoal)

Male:
- Discharge of Prostatic fluid at stool.
- Itching and moisture at Thighs near Scrotum.

Female:
- Premature and Too Copious Menses.
- Discharge of Pale Blood
- Vulva: Swollen, Apthae, Varices on pudenda.
- Leucorrhoea: Before Menses, is Thick, Greenish,
- Milky and Excoriating.
- Burning in Hands and Soles, during Menstruation.

76. CARBOLICUM ACIDUM
(Carbolic Acid-Phenol)

Male:
- Irritable bladder.
- Frequent Urination at Night in Old men.
- Prostatic hyperplasis and diabetes.

Female:
- Discharge always offensive.
- Pustules around vulva containing bloody pus.
- Agonising Backache, across Loin with dragging down thighs.
- Pain in Left Ovary: Worse: Walking in Open Air.
- Cervical erosion: Foetid, Acrid Discharge.
- Leucorrhoea in young Girls.
- Puerperal Fever with Offensive Discharge.
- Irritating Leucorrhoea causing itching and burning.

Useful in:

Male:
- Irritable Bladder
- Benign Prostatic Hyperplasia

Female:
- Backache
- Leucorrhoea
- Cervical Erosion

77. CARBONIUM SULPHURATUM
(Bisulphide of Carbon)

Male:

- Impotence
- Desire lost.
- Parts: atrophied.
- Frequent profuse emissions.
- Plumbism.
- Peripheral Neuritis.
- Very useful in patients those who, broken down by abuse of alcohol.
- Lack of Vital Heat.

Useful in:
Male:

- Erectile Dysfunction
- Impotence
- Atrophy of the Testes

78. CARCINOSIN
(A Nosode from Carcinoma)

Female:
- Carcinoma of Mammary Gland.
- Great Pain.
- Indurations of the Glands of Uterus.
- Offensive Discharge.
- Haemorrhage and Burning Pain.

Useful in:
Female:
- Carcinoma of Breast.

79. CAULOPHYLLUM
(Blue Cohosh)

Female:

- Extra ordinary Rigidity of Os Uterii.
- Severe spasmodic pain, fly in all directions.
- Shivering without progress-False pain.
- Revives: Labour Pain and further progress of Labour.
- After Pains.
- Leucorrhoea with Moth-Spots on forehead.
- Habitual Abortion from Uterine Debility.
- Needle like pain in Cervix.
- Dysmenorrhoea-with pain, flying to other parts of body.
- Lochia: Protracted. Great Atony.
- Menses and Leucorrhoea: both profuse.

Useful in:
Female:

- Dysmenorrhoea
- Leucorrhoea
- Habitual Abortion
- Rigidity of Uterine Os
- Uterine Inertia
- Atony of Uterus

80. CAUSTICUM.

(Hahnemann's Tincture Acris sine Kali)

Female:

- Uterine inertia during Labour.
- Menses: Ceases at Night. Flow only during day.
- Leucorrhoea at night with great weakness.
- Menses: Delayed, Late.

81. CENCHRIS CONTORTRIX
Ancistrodon (Copperhead Snake)

Female:
- Increased Sexual Desire
- Pain: at Right Ovarian Region.

82. CHAMOMILLA
(German Chamomile)

Female:

- Uterine Haemorrhages.
- Profuse discharge of clotted, dark blood with labour like pain.
- Labour pains: Spasmodic, Pressing Upwards.
- Intolerant of pain.
- Breasts: Nipples inflamed, Tender to touch
- Infant's breast : tender
- Leucorrhoea: Yellow and acrid.

83. CHELIDONIUM MAJUS
(Celandine)

Male:
- Serous Effusion
- Hydrocele.

Female:
- Menses: Too late and Too profuse.

84. CHIMAPHILA UMBELLATA
(Pipsissewa)

Male:

- Smarting in Urethra from neck of Bladder to Urethral Meatus.
- Gleet.
- Loss of Prostatic Fluid.
- Prostatic Enlargement and Irritation.

Female:

- Labia: Inflamed and Swollen.
- Pain in Vagina.
- Hot flushes.
- Breasts: Painful Tumours of Mammae.
- Not ulcerated with undue secretion of milk.
- Rapid Atrophy of Breast.
- Women with very large breasts, having Tumours in the
- Mammary Gland with sharp pain through it.

85. CIMEX ACANTHIA
(Bed Bug)

Female:

- Shooting pain from vagina up, towards Left Ovary.

86. CIMICIFUGA RACEMOSA
(Black Snake Root)

Female:

- Amenorrhoea
- Pain in Ovarian Region-Shoots upwards and down, towards anterior surface of Thighs.
- Pain, immediately before menses
- Menses: Profuse, Dark, Coagulated, and Offensive with Backache.
- Menses: Always irregular.
- Nervousness
- Ovarian Neuralgia.
- Pain across pelvis, from Hip to Hip.
- After Pains: with great sensitiveness and intolerance of pain.
- Breasts: Infra-mammary Pains: Worse on left side.
- Facial Blemishes in Young Girls and Women.

87. CINA
(Worm Seed)

Female:

- Uterine Haemorrhage before Puberty.

88. CINCHONA OFFICINALIS.

(Peruvian Bark-China)

Male:

- Debility from Exhausting discharges.
- Loss of Vital Fluids.
- Nervous Erethism.
- Excited, lascivious fancy.
- Frequent Emissions, followed by great weakness.
- Orchitis.

Female:

- Menses: Too early, associated with.....
- Dark clots and abdominal Distension.
- Profuse menses with pain.
- Desire: Too strong.
- Bloody Leucorrhoea-seems to take the place of the usual menstrual discharge
- Painful Heaviness in pelvis.

89. CINNABARIS
MERCURIUS SULPHURATUS RUBER
(Mercuric Sulphide)

Male:

- Warts on prepuce, Swollen and Bleeds easily.
- Testicles: Enlarged.
- Buboes.
- Angry looking chancres.
- Syphilides: Squamous and Vesicular.

Female:

- Leucorrhoea.
- Feeling of pressure in Vagina.

90. CINNAMONIUM
(Cinnamon)

Female:

- Bearing down sensation.
- Menses: Early, Profuse, Prolonged, Bright Red.
- Sleepy
- No desire for anything.
- Fingers seem swollen.
- Uterine Haemorrhages caused by—over lifting during Puerperal state.
- Menorrhagia.
- Cancer: Where pain and Offensive odour present.

91. CLEMATIS ERECTA.
(Virgin's Bower)

Male:

- Ileo-caecal Neuralgia.
- Testicles: Indurated with bruised feeling.
- Swelling of Scrotum: Right half only.
- Orchitis.
- All complains from suppressed Gonorrhoea.
- Violent erections with stitches in Urethra.
- Testicles: Hang heavy or retracted, along with Pain in Spermatic Cord - Worse: Right Side.

92. COBALTUM
(The metal-Cobalt)

Male:

- Pain in Right Testicle
- Pain: Relieves: After Urinating.
- Emissions without Erections.
- Impotence.
- Backache in Lumbar Region with weak legs.
- Lewd Dreams.
- Pain in end of Urethra: with Greenish Discharge.
- Brown Spots on Genitals and Abdomen.

93. COCCULUS
(Indian Cockle)

Female:

This medicine shows a special affinity and attraction for,

- Light haired females, esp. during Pregnancy, causing much
- Nausea and Backache.
- Un-married and Childless Women.
- Sensitive and Romantic Girls
- Dysmenorrhoea: with profuse, dark menses.
- Menses: Too early, clotted and associated with Spasmodic Colic.
- Painful pressing in Uterine Region, followed by Haemorrhoids.
- Leucorrhoea: Purulent, Gushing, between Menses, very weakening, can hardly and scarcely speak.
- Very weak during Menstruation, scarcely able to stand.

94. COCCUS CACTI
(Cochineal)

Female:
- Menses: Too early, Too Profuse, Black and Thick.
- Dark Clots with Dysuria.
- Intermittent Menstruation.
- Menstrual Flow: Only in evening and at night.
- Large clots escape while urinating.
- Labia: Inflamed.

95. COFFEA CRUDA
(Unroasted Coffee)

Female:

- Menses: Too early and long lasting.
- Dysmenorrhoea.
- Large clots of black blood.
- Hypersensitive Vulva and Vagina.
- Voluptuous Itching.

96. COLCHICUM
(Meadow Saffron)

Female:
- Pruritus of Genitals.
- Cold feeling in thighs after Menstrual period.
- Sensation of swelling in Vulva and Clitoris.
- Always great prostration.
- Complete Mental and Physical exhaustion.

97. COLLINSONIA CANADENSIS
(Stone Root)

Remarkable effect on pelvic and portal congestion which results in piles and constipation.

Female:

- Dysmenorrhoea – pruritus of Vulva
- Prolapse of uterus
- Swelling and Dark Redness of Genitals; which causes Pain on Sitting down.
- Membranous Dysmenorrhoea; with Constipation.
- Cold feeling in thighs after menstruation.
- Sensation of Swelling of Labia and Clitoris.

98. COLOCYNTHIS
(Bitter Cucumber)
Ideal for...
Women with copious menstruation and patient having
sedentary habits

Female:
- Burning pain in Ovary.
- Must draw up double, with great Restlessness.
- Round, small cystic tumours in Ovaries or Broad ligaments.
- Wants abdomen supported by pressure.
- Bearing down Cramps, causing her to bend double.
- Patient feels better: by doubling up, Hard Pressure, Warmth, Lying with head bent forward.

99. CONIUM
(PIOSON HEMLOCK)

Male:
- Desire Increased
- Power Decreased
- Sexual Nervousness with feeble erection
- Effect of Suppressed Sexual Appetite
- Testicles: Hard and Enlarged

Female:
- Dysmenorrhoea with drawing down thighs
- Mammae: Lax and Shrunken – Hard.
- Breasts: Painful to touch – Stitches in Nipples.
- Wants to press Breast hard with Hands.
- **Menses** Delayed and scanty – Parts sensitive.
  - Breasts Enlarge and become Painful during and after menses.
  - Rash before menses.
  - Itching around Pudenda.
  - Unready conception.
  - Indurations of Ext. Os and Cervix.
- **Ovaritis:**
  - Ovary enlarged, indurated, Lancinating Pain.
  - Ill effects of Repressed Sexual desire or suppressed Menses, or from excessive indulgence.
  - Leucorrhoea after urination.

100. CONVALLARIA MAJALIS
(Lily of the Valley)

Female:
- Great soreness in Uterine Region; with sympathetic palpitation of heart.
- Pain in Sacro – Iliac Joints, running down legs.
- Itching at Urinary Meatus and Vaginal Orifice.

101. COPAIVA
(Balsam of Copaiva)

Act powerful on mucus membranes.

Male:

- Testicles: sensitive and swollen.

Female:

- Itching of Vulva and Anus; with Bloody, Purulent discharge
- Profuse, strong – smelling menstrual discharge with Pains radiating to hipbones with Nausea.

102. CORALLIUM
(Red Coral)

Male:

- Ulcers on Glans and inner prepuce; with yellow ichor.
- Emissions and weakened sexual power.
- Profuse perspiration of Genitals.

103. COTYLEDON

(Penay Wort)

Female

- Breast:
  - Pain under Left Nipple – Aching in Right Breast.
  - Pain through to Scapula from region of Left Breast.
  - Pain at angles of scapulae.
  - Full Bursting feeling, as if from obstruction at heart.
  - Chocking fullness in Throat.
  - Breathing Oppressed.

104. CROCUS SATIVA
(Saffron)

Female:
- Threatened Abortion.
- When Haemorrhage is dark and stringy.
- Urging of Blood to genitals.
- Menses: dark, Viscid, too frequent and Copious.
- Black and Slimy.
- Uterine Haemorrhage....clots with long strings.
- Worse: from least movement.
- Jerking Pain in Interior of Left Breast, as if drawn towards back by means of Thread.
- A bounding feeling, as if something alive in Right Breast.

105. CROTALUS HORRIDUS
(Rattle Snake)

Female:

- Prolonged Menses. Dysmenorrhoea.
- Pain extends down thighs, with aching in region of heart.
- Uterine Haemorrhages with faintness at Stomach.
- Puerperal Fever; Offensive Lochia.
- Phlegmasia Alba dolens.
- Sensation as though uterine would drop out.
- Painful drawing in uterine ligaments.
- Cannot keep legs still.

106. CUBEBA

Effective on Mucus Membranes generally especially UTI

- Leucorrhoea: in little girls.

107. CUPRUM ARSENICUM

Male:
- Perspiration of scrotum.
- Scrotum is constantly damp and moist.
- Boils on scrotum.
- Purulent discharge of a white colour from Urethra.
- Tingling and Burning in Urethra.
- Pain in Prostate.
- Pain in Penis.

108. CUPRUM METALLICUM
(Copper-The Metal)

Female:

- Menses: Too late, Protracted.
- Cramps, extending into chest, before, during and after suppression of Menses.
- Also from suppressed foot sweat.
- Ebullition of blood; Palpitation.
- Chlorosis, After Pains.

109. CURARE - WOORARI
(Arrow Poison)

Female:

- Dysmenorrhoea.
- Menses Too Early.
- Colic during Menses.
- Headache, Kidney Pain.
- Leucorrhoea – Thick, Purulent, Offensive.

110. CYCLAMEN
(Sow - bread)

Female:

- Menses profuse, black, membranous, clotted.
- Too early with Labour like Pains from back to Pubes. Flow less when moving about.
- Menstrual Irregularities with Migraine and Blindness.
- Fiery spots before eyes.
- Hiccough during Pregnancy.
- Post – Partum Haemorrhage with colicky bearing down Pains, with relief after gush of blood.
- After Menses, swelling of Breasts with Milky secretion.

111. DIGITALIS

(Fox glove)

Male:

- Nightly Emission with great weakness of Genitals after coitus.
- Hydrocele.
- Scrotum: Enlarged like a Bladder.
- Gonorrhoea - Balantitis(Inflammation of Glans Penis) with,
- Oedema of Prepuce.
- Dropsical Swelling of Genitals.
- Enlarged Prostate.
- Prostatitis.

Female:

- Labour like Pains in Abdomen and back before menses. Uterine Haemorrhage.

112. DIOSCOREA VILLOSA
(Wild Yam)

Male:
- Relaxation and Coldness of Organs.
- Pain shoots into Testicles from region of kidneys.
- Strong smelling sweat on scrotum and Pubes.
- Emission in sleep as from sexual Atony; with weak knees.

Female:
- Uterine Colic.
- Pain radiates from Uterus.
- Vivid Dreams.

113. DIOSMA LINCARIS
(BUKU - from Cape of Good Hope)

Female:

- Hysteria – Convulsion
- Useful in Haematuria with…
    - Ovarian Lesion
    - Uterine Lesion

114. DULCAMARA
(Bitter Sweet)

Female:

- Suppression of Menses from cold or Dampness.
- Before appearance of Menses, a rash appears on skin or sexual Excitement.
- Dysmenorrhoea: White blotches all over.
- Mammae engorged and sore, delicate, sensitive to cold

115. ECHINACEA - RUDBECKIA
(Purple Cone Flower)

Female:

- Puerperal Septicaemia.
- Discharges Suppressed.
- Abdomen sensitive and Tympanitic.
- Leucorrhoea: Offensive, excoriating

116. ERIGERON – LEPTILON CANADENSE

(Fleabane)

Haemorrhages are caused and cured by this Remedy.

Female:

- Metrorrhagia with violent Irritation of Rectum and Bladder; and Prolapsus Uteri.
- Bright – Red flow. Menorrhagia, profuse Leucorrhoea.
- Bloody Lochia Returns after least motion; comes in gushes, between Periods.
- Leucorrhoea with urinary irritation.
- PREGNANT Women with "weak Uterus".
- A bloody discharge on slightest excretion.
- Bleeding Piles.
- Nose bleed instead of menses
- Vicarious Menses

117. ERIODICTYOM
(Yerba Santa)

Male:

- Sore, Dragging in Testicle.
- Could not bear any Pressure around Genitals, more than gentle support.

118. ERYNGIUM AQUATICUM
(Button Snake Root)

Male:

- Discharge of Prostatic Fluid from slight causes.
- Seminal Emissions without Erections with Lassitude.

119. EUCALYPTUS GLOBULUS
(Blue Gum Tree)

Very Powerful Anti -Septic

Female:

- Leucorrhoea: Acrid – Foetid.
- Ulcer around Orifice of Urethra.

120. EUPATORIUM PURPUREUM
(Queen of the Meadow)

Impotency and Sterility

Female
- Pain around Left Ovary
- Threatened Abortion
- External Genitals feels as if wet.

121. EUPHORBIA LATHYRIS
(Gopher plant – Caper Spurge)

Male:

- Inflammation of scrotum resulting in deep, acrid ulcers, with intense itching and burning.

- Worse: Touching the parts from Washing.

122. EUPHRASIA
(Eye - Bright)

Male:

- Spasmodic Retraction of the Genitals with Pressure above Pubic bone.
- Condyloma
- Sycotic Excrescences.
- Prostatitis.
- Nocturnal Irritability of Bladder.
- Dribbling Urine.

Female:

- Menses: Painful
- Flow last only an HOUR or Day
- Late, scanty, short.
- Amenorrhoea with Opthalmia.

123. EUPION
(Wood Tar Distillation)

Female:

- Remedy for Uterine Displacement.
- Pain in Back, followed by a Bland Leucorrhoea
- Menses: Too early and copious – Flow remains thin.
- Burning in Right Ovary.
- Gushing Leucorrhoea
- Chronic Tubal Disease
- Uterine Flexions.
- During Menses: Irritable Stitches in chest and Heart.
- After Menses, yellow Leucorrhoea with severe Backache.
- When Pain in Back ceases, the discharge gushes out.
- Sore Pain between Labia during Urination.
- Pruritus Pudendi.
- Labia Swollen.

124. FAGOPYRUM

(Buckwheat)

Female:
- Pruritus Vulvae with yellow Leucorrhoea.
- Worse Rest.
- Burning in Right Ovary.

125. FERRUM IODATUM
(Iodide of Iron)

Female:
- On sitting feels as if something pressed upwards in Vagina.
- Much Bearing Down.
- Uterine Displacements.
- Retro version and Prolapse of Uterus.
- Leucorrhoea like Boiled starch.
- Menses: Suppressed or scanty.
- Itching and soreness of vulva and vagina.

126. FERRUM METALLICUM
(Iron)

Female:

- Menses Remit a Day or Two and then it returns.
- Discharge of Long piece from Uterus.
- Women who are weak, delicate chlorotic yet have a fiery Red Face.
- Menses: Too Early, Too Profuse, Last too long, Pale, watery.
- Sensitive Vagina.
- Tendency to Abortion.
- Prolapse of Vagina.

127. FERRUM PHOSPHORICUM
(Phosphate of Iron)

Female:

- Menses every three weeks; with bearing down sensation and Pain on top of Head.
- Vaginismus.
- Vagina: Dry and Hot.

128. FERRUM PICRICUM
(Picrate of Iron)

Male:

- Senile Hypertrophy of PROSTATE.
- Smarting at the Neck of Bladder and Penis.

129. FLUORICUM ACIDUM
(Hydrofluoric Acid)

Male:

- Burning in Urethra.
- Sexual Passion and desire increased with erection at night, during sleep.
- Swollen scrotum.

Female:

- Menses Copious, frequent, too long.
- Ulceration of Uterus and External os,
- Cervical Erosion
- Copious and Excoriating Leucorrhoea.
- Nymphomania

130. FORMICA RUFA (MYRMEXINE)
(Crushed Live Ants)

Male:

- Seminal Emissions,
- Weakness "Slothful to Venery"

131. FRAXINUS AMERICANA
(White Ash)

Female:

- Uterus enlarged and Patulous.
- Watery un-irritating Leucorrhoea. Bland Discharge.
- Fibroid with bearing down sensation.
- Cramping in feet.
- Worse in afternoon and night.
- Dysmenorrhoea

132. GULTHERIA
(Winter Green)

- Cystic and Prostatic irritation.
- Undue Sexual Excitement.
- Renal Inflammation.

133. GELSEMIUM
(Yellow Jasmine)

Male:

- Spermatorrhoea without Erection.
- Genitals cold and Relaxed.
- Scrotum continuously sweating. Sweat in palms and Soles
- Gonorrhoea - first stage, Discharge: scanty.
- Tendency to corrode.
- Little pain but much Heat.
- Smarting at Meatus.

Female:

- Rigid External Os – Sensation as if uterus were squeezed.
- Vaginismus – False Labour Pain.
- Pain passes up back.
- Dymenorrhoea with scanty flow.
- Menses: Retarded.
- Pain extends to back and hips.
- Aphonia and sore throat during Menses.

134. GERANIUM MACULATUM
(Crane's Bill)

Female:
- Menses: Too Profuse
- PPH: Postpartum Haemorrhage
- sore nipples

135. GINSENG

Male:

- Rheumatic Pains after frequent emission.
- Weakness of Genital organs.
- Voluptuous tickling at the end of Urethra.
- Sexual Excitement.
- Pressure in Testicles.

136. GLONOINE
(Nitro Glycerine)

Female:

- Menses: delayed or sudden cessation with congestion to head.
- Climectric flushing.
- Menopausal syndrome.

137. GLYCERINUM

Female:

- Profuse, long-lasting flow with bearing down Heaviness in uterus.
- General sense of exhaustion.

138. GNAPHALIUM
(Cud Weed) Old Balsam

- Prominent Remedy for Sciatica
- Prominent Remedy for Sacro-Iliac Strain
- Pain is associated with Numbness.

Female:

- Weight and Fullness in Pelvis.
- Dysmenorrhoea with scanty and Painful menses.

139. GOSSYPIUM
(Cotton Plant)

- Powerful Emmenagogue.
- Disturbed Uterine Function and Pregnancy.
- It Relieves: Tardy menses, especially with sensation that the flow is about to start and yet does not do so.

Female:

- Labia swollen and itching...intermittent Pain in Ovaries.
- Retained Placenta.
- Tumour of the Breast with swelling of axillary glands.
- Morning sickness with sensitive Uterine Region.
- Suppressed Menstruation.
- Menses: Too watering.
- Backache... Weight and dragging in Pelvis.
- Sub involution of Uterus.
- Uterine fibroids with Gastric Pain and Debility.

140. GRAPHITIS
(Black Lead - Plumbago)

Anti – Psoric of a great power. Pt. is stout, fair and constipated

Constitution:

- Fat, Chilly and Costive with Delayed Menstrual History. Catches cold easily.
- Tendency to Skin affection.

Male:

- Sexual Debiltiy with Increased desire
- Aversion to coition
- Too early or no ejaculation.
- Herpetic eruption on Organs.

Female:

- Menses: Too late with constipation.
- Pale and scanty with tearing pain in epigastrium and itching before.
- Hoarseness, coryza, cough, sweats and morning sickness during menstruation.
- Leucorrhoea: Pale, thin Profuse, white, excoriating with great weakness in Back.
- Breast: Swollen and hard. Induration.
- Nipples sore, cracked a Blistered.
- Induration of Ovaries, Uterus and Mamme.
- Decided Aversion to coitus

141. GRATIOLA
(Hedge Hyssop)

Female:

- Nymphomania
- Menses: Too Profuse, Premature and Too long.
- Leucorrhoea and
- Gonorrhoea.

142. GAUCO
(Mikania - Climbing Hemp Weed)

Female:

- Leucorrhoea – copious, corroding, putrid and debilitating.
- Itching and smarting at night, as if fire were running out of parts.

143. GUAIACUM
(Resin of Lignum Vitae)

Female:

- Ovaritis in Rheumatic Patient with irregular menstruation and Dysmenorrhoea.
- Irritable Bladder.

144. HAEMATOXYLON
(Logwood)

Female:

- Pain in Hypogastrium attended with slimy whitish Leucorrhoea.
- Weak feeling with Painful bearing down sensation at Menstrual Period.

145. HAMAMELIS VIRGINICA
(Witch Hazel)

Venous congestion – Haemorrhage – varicose veins and haemorrhoids with bruised soreness of affected parts.

Male:
- Pain in spermatic cord, running into testes.
- Varicocele
- Pain in Testicles: Orchitis
- Testicles enlarged, hot and Painful.
- Epididymitis.

Female:

- Ovarian Congestion and Neuralgia.
- Feel very sore.
- Vicarious Menstruation.
- Uterine Haemorrhage with bearing down Pain in back.
- Menses: Dark, Profuse with soreness in abdomen.
- Metrorrhagia occurring midway between menstrual Periods, with intermenstrual Pain.
- Vagina very Tender.
- Profuse Leucorrhoea.
- Vulva itches.
- Milk – leg, haemorrhoids, and sore nipples after confinement.
- Metrorrhagia, Passive flow.
- Vaginismus, Ovaritis, Soreness over the whole Abdomen.
- Phlegmasia Alba.

146. HEDEOMA
(Penny Royal)

Female symptoms are more marked; with Nervous Disturbances.

Female:

- Bearing down pains with much Backache.
- Less by least movement.
- Leucorrhoea with itching and burning.
- Ovaries Congested and Painful.
- Bearing down spasmodic contractions.

Concomtant:

- Red Sand in Urine Pain along Ureter.

147. HELLEBORUS
(Snow Rose)

Female:

- Sensorial Depression.
- Muscular Weakness.
- Involuntary Sighing.
- Complete Unconsciousness.
- Picks Lips and Clothes.
- Horrible smell from mouth.(Foetar Oris)

148. HELONIAS - CHAMAELIRIUM
(Unicorn Root)

Tired, Back achy Female, with great languor and prostration; with weakness.
Dragging in the Sacrum and Weight in the Pelvis

Female:

- Dragging in the sacral region with Prolapse especially after a miscarriage.
- Prurtius Vulvae.
- Backache after miscarriage.
- Weight and soreness in womb.
- Consciousness of uterus.
- Menses: Too Frequent, Too profuse.
- Leucorrhoea.
- Breasts: Swollen, Nipples Painful and Tender.
- Parts: Hot, Red, Swollen, Burns and itch terribly.
- Albuminuria: during Pregnancy.
- Debility attending the Menopause.

149. HEPAR SULPHURIS CALCAREUM
(Calcium Sulphide: Proved by Hahnemann)

- Great sensitiveness to all impressions.
- Tendency to Suppuration.

Male:

- Herpes, sensitive, bleed easily.
- Ulcers externally on prepuce and similar to chancre. (Nit acid).
- Excitement and emission without amorous fancies.
- Itching of Glands, Franum and Scrotum.
- Suppurating Inguinal Glands.
- Figwarts of offensive odour.
- Humid soreness on genitals and between scrotum and thighs.
- Obstinate gonorrhoea - "Does Not Get Well"

Female:

- Discharge of Blood form Uterus.
- Itching of Pudenda and Nipples, worse during Menses.
- Menses: Late and scanty
- Abscesses of Labiae with great sensitiveness. Extremely sensitive
- Leucorrhoea "Smells like old cheese" (Sanicula)
- Profuse perspiration at the climacteric (Tilla, Jaborandi)

150. HIPPOMANES
(A Meconium deposit out of the Amniotic Fluid taken from the Colt)

- Old Famous Aphrodisiacum of the Greek authors.

Male:
- Sexual Desire Increased.
- Prostatitis
- Drawing Pain in Testicles.

151. HIPPURIC ACID

Female:

- Menstrual Blood Flow for three weeks with complete relief of muscular and Joint Pains

152. HYDRASTIS
(Golden Seal)

- Goitre of Puberty and Pregnancy.

Male:
- Gonorrhoea, second stage, discharge thick and yellow.

Female:
- Erosion and Excoriation of Cervix.
- Leucorrhoea, worse after Menses. (Bov, calc. Carb) acid and corroding, shreddy, tenacious.
- Menorrhagia.
- Pruritus vulvae with Profuse Leucorrhoea.
- Sexual excitement.
- Tumours of Breast, Nipples Retracted.

153. HYDROCOTYLE
(Indian Penny Wort)

- Of great use in ulceration of womb.
- Pains of cervical cancer.

Female:
- Prucitus of Vagina.
- Inflammation of neck of Bladder.
- Heat within Vagina.
- Granular Ulceration of womb.
- Prefuse Leucorrhoea.
- Dull pain in ovarian region.
- Cervical Redness.

154. HYDROPHOBINUM
(Lyssin – saliva of Rabid Dog)

- Complains from abnormal Sexual Desire.

Male:
- Lascivious; Priapism with frequent emissions.
- No emissions during coition.
- Atrophy of Testicles.
- Complains from abnormal Sexual Desire.

Female:
- Uterine sensitiveness, concious of womb (Helon)
- Feels Prolapsed.
- Vagina sensitive, rendering coition Painful.
- Uterine displacement.

155. HYOSCYAMUS
(Henbane)

Male:
- Impotence. Lascivious; exposes his person.
- Plays with genitals during fever.

Female:

- Before Menses, Hysterical spasms.
- Excited sexual desire.
- During Menses, convulsive movements.
- Urinary reflux and sweat.
- Lochia suppressed.
- Spasms of Pregnant women.
- Puerperal mania.

156. HYPERICUM
(St. John's Wort)

- Relieve Pain after surgery.
- Spasms after every injury.
- Coccygodynia. (Bachache)

157. ICHTHYOLUM

- Anti – Parastic
- Uric Acid Diathesis
- Chronic Hives
- Aids (Helps) Nutrition

Female:

- Fullness in Lower Abdomen.
- Nausea at time of Menses

158. IGNATIA
(St. Ignatius Bean)

- **Female Remedy.**
- Emotional Element is upper most and co-ordination of function is interfered with Tendency to clonic spasm.

Mind:

- Changeable mood
- Adapted to Nervous Temperament.
- Very Sensitive, Melancholic, Sad, tearful
- Easily excited nature.
- Dark, Mild disposition.
- Quick to Perceive – Rapid in Execution.
- Sudden change of emotional and physical condition. Silent brooding.
- Great contradiction
- Alert
- Nervous – apprehensive
- Sighing and sobbing.
- Coffee aggravates
- Tabbacco aggravates.
- Bad effects of grief.
- Menses: Black, Too early - Too Profuse or Scanty
- Menses: associated with Spasmodic Pain in Stomach and Abdomen with languor.
- Sexual Frigidity.
- Suppression of Emotions from grief.

159. INDIUM
(Metal Indium)

Male:

- Horribly Offensive smell of Urine.
- Emissions too Frequent.
- Diminished Power
- Testicles Tender
- Drawing Pains along spermatic card
- Sexual Psychopathy.

160. INULA
(Scabwort)

Female:

- Menses: Too early and Painful
- Labour like Pains
- Urging to Stool, dragging in genitals with Violent Backache.
- Itching of Legs during Menses.
- Chattering of teeth from cold during Menses.
- Moving about in Abdomen, Stitches in genitals.
- Chronic Metritis.

161. IODUM
(Iodine)

General:
- Great Appetite but Loss Of Flesh
- Great debility, the slightest efforts induces perspiration.

Constitution:
- Thin, dark complexioned with enlarged Lymphatic glands.
- Tendency for: Acute Exacerbation of Chronic Inflammation.
- Acts on Connective Tissue.

Mind:
- "Anxiety when quite".

Male:
- Testicles swollen and indurated.
- Hydrocele
- Loss of sexual Power…with testicular atrophy.

Female:
- Great weakness during Menses.
- Irregular Menses.
- Uterine Haemorrhage
- DUB(Dysfunctional Uterine Bleeding)
- Ovaritis
- Wedge – like Pain from ovary to Uterus.
- Dwindling of Mammary glands.
- Nodositis in skin of Mammae.
- Acrid Leucorrhoea - Thick and Slimy
- Wedge - like Pain in Right Ovarian Region.

162. IPECACUANHA
(Ipecac Root)

- Persistent Nausea...with Clean Tongue and much saliva.
- Profuse and Bright Red Haemorrhage.
- Amoebic Dysentery.

Female:

- Uterine Haemorrhage...Profuse, Bright, Gushing with constant Nausea.
- Vomiting during Pregnancy. (Hyper emesis Gravidarum)
- Pain from Navel to Uterus.
- Menses too early and too Profuse.

163. JACARANDA
(Brazilian Caroba Tree)

- Indicated in Venereal diseases
- Morning Sickness.

Male:

- Urinary: Urethra Inflamed
- Heat and Pain in Penis
- Painful erections
- Phimosis
- Prepuce Painful and swollen
- Chancroid
- Chordee
- Itching Pimples on glans and Prepuce.

164. JONOSIA ASOCA
(Bark of Indian Ashoka Tree)

- Amenorrhoea
- Metrorrhagia

  - Delayed and Irregular Menses
  - Menstrual Colic
  - Amenorrhoea
  - Pain in Ovaries before flow
  - Menorrhagia
  - Irritable Bladder
  - Leucorrhoea

165. KALI ARSENICUM
(Fowler's Solution)

Tendency for malignancy.

Female:

- Cauliflower excrescence of OS Uteri.
- With flying Pains.
- With foul smelling discharge and Pressure below Pubis.

166. KALI BICHROMICUM
(Bichromate of Potash)

Male:
- Itching and Pain of Penis, with Pustules.
- Ulcers with Paroxysmal stitches, more at night.
- Constriction at Root of Penis, at night on awakening.
- Syphilitic Ulcers, with cheesy tenacious exudation.

Female:
- Yellow, tenacious Leucorrhoea,
- Pruritus of vulva with great Burning and excitement.
- Prolapsus Uteri, worse in hot weather.

167. KALI BROMATUM
(Bromide of Potash)

Male:
- Debility and impotence
- Bad effects of Sexual Excess, resulting in loss of memory and impaired co-ordination.
- Numbness and tingling in limbs.
- Sexual Excitement during partial Slumber.

Female:

- Pruritus
- Ovarian Neuralgia with great nervous uneasiness.
- Exaggerated Sexual Desire.
- Cystic tumours of Ovaries.

168. KALI CARBONICUM
(Carbonate of Potassium)

Male:

- Complains from coition.
- Deficient Sexual instinct.
- Excessive Emissions followed by Weakness.

Female:
- Menses: Early, Profuse or too late, Pale and scanty with soreness about genitalia.
- Pain from back Pass down through gluteal muscles with cutting in abdomen.
- Pain through left labium, extending through abdomen to chest.
- Delayed Menses in young girls with chest symptoms or ascitis.
- Difficult first Menses.
- Complains after Parturition.
- Uterine Haemorrhages, constant oozing after copious flow, with violent Backache, relieved by sitting and pressure.

169. KALI SALICYLICUM

Vomiting of Pregnancy

170. KALI MURIATICUM

Female:

- Menses: Too late or suppressed, checked or too early.
- Excessive Discharge.
- Dark, clotted or tough, black blood like TAR. (Platina)
- Leucorrhoea:
  Discharge of milky white mucus thick,
  Non- irritating, bland.
- Morning Sickness: With vomiting of white phlegm.
- Breasts: Bunches in Breast feel quite soft and are tender.

171. KALI NITRICUM - NITRUM
(Nitrate of Potassium - Saltpeter)

Female:

- Menses: Too early, profuse, black.
- Proceeded and with violent Backache.
- Leucorrhoea: Burning Pains in the ovarian region only during menses.

172. KALI PHOSPHORICUM
(Phosphate of Potassium)

Best Nerve Remedy. "Want of Nerve Power"

Male:
- Nocturnal Emissions
- Sexual Power diminished
- Prostrations after coitus. (Kali Carb)

Female:
- Menstruation too late or too scanty in Pale, irritable, sensitive, lachrymose females.
- Too profuse discharge, deep red or blackish – red, thin and not coagulating; sometimes with offensive odour.
- Feeble and ineffectual Labour Pain.

173. KALI SULPHURICUM
(Potassium Sulphate)

Male:

- Gonorrhoea; discharge slimy, yellowish – green.
- Orchitis, Gleet.

Female:

- Menses: too late, scanty with feeling of weight in Abdomen, Metrorrhagia.

174. KALMIA LATIFOLIA
(Mountain Laurel)

Female:
- Menses too early or suppressed with Pain in Limbs and back and inside of thighs.
- Leucorrhoea follows Menses.

175. KREOSOTUM
(Beechwood Kreosote)

Female:

- Corrosive itching within vulva.
- Burning and swelling of Labia.
- Violent itching between Labia and thighs.
- During Menses, difficult hearing.
- Buzzing and Roaring eruptions after.
- Burning and soreness in external and internal parts
- Leucorrhoea: Yellow acrid, odour of green corn, worst between Periods.
- Haemorrhage after coition.
- Menses: Too early, Prolonged.
- Vomiting of Pregnancy with Ptyalism.
- Menstrual flow: intermits (like pulsatilla) ceases on sitting or walking,
- Re-appears on lying down.
- Pain worse after menses.
- Lochia: Offensive and Intermits.

176. LAC CANINUM

(Dog's Milk)

Female:

- Menses: too early, profuse, flow in gushes.
- Breasts: swollen.
- Painful before (Calc. C; Con; Puls) Menses.
- Breasts: better on appearance of Menses.
- Mastitis: worse, least jar.
- Helps to dry up Milk, Who cannot nurse baby.
- Sinking at Epigastrium.
- Sexual Organs easily excited.
- Backache: Spine, very sensitive to touch or pressure.
- Galactorrhoea.

177. LACHESIS
(Bush master or Surucucu)

Female:

- Menopausal or Climectric troubles.
- Palpitation.
- Flushes of Heat with Haemorrhage.
- Vertex Headache.
- Fainting Spell… Syncopeal Feelings
- Worse by pressure or clothes. Can't bear tight clothing around Neck.
- Menses: Too short, too feeble, Pains all relieved by the flow (Eupion).
- Left Ovary: Very Painful and Swollen and indurated.
- Breasts: Mammae inflamed, bluish.
- Back: Coccyx and Sacrum Pain especially on rising from sitting posture.
- Acts especially very well at the beginning and stoppage or closure of menstruation.

178. LACTUCA VIROSA
(Acid Lettuce)

Female:
- Promotes Catamania
- Increases Milk in Breasts. (Asafoetida)
- Good Galactogogue.

179. LAPPA ARCTIUM
(Burdock)

Female:

- Uterine Displacement, Prolapse of Uterus
- An exceedingly sore, bruised feeling in uterus with great relaxation of vaginal tissues.
- Apparently entire Lack of Tonicity of Pelvic Contents.
- These symptoms all aggravated by standing, walking, a mis-step, or sudden jar.

180. LECITHIN

Male:
- Male sexual power lost or enfeebled.
- Anaphrodisia means lack of sexual Desire.

Female:

- Ovarian Insufficiency.

181. LILIUM TIGRINUM
(Tiger Lily)

- Powerful influence over the Pelvic Organs.
- Best indicated to Unmarried women.

Female:

- Menses: Early, scanty, dark, clotted, offensive.
- Flow only when moving about.
- Bearing down sensation with urgent desire for stool; as though all organs would escape.
- Prolapse of uterus and Arteversion
- Constant desire to support parts externally.
- Pain in ovaries and down thighs.
- Acrid brown Leucorrhoea; smarting in Labia.
- Sexual Instinct awakened.
- Bloated feeling in uterine region.
- Subinvolution.
- Pruritus Pudendi.

182. LUPULUS - HUMLUS
(Hops)

Male:

- Painful Erection. Emissions, depending on sexual weakness and after onanism.
- Spearmatorrhoea. Giddiness and Stupefecation.
- Lupulin 1x trit: > Best in seminal Emissions

183. LYCOPODIUM
(Club Moss)

Male:
- No Erectile Power
- Impotence.
- Premature emissions. (Calad; Selen; Agnus.)
- Enlarged Prostate
- Condylomata.

Female:

- Menses too late; last too long, too profuse.
- Vagina: Dry
- Painful Intercourse.
- Pain: Right Ovarian Region.
- Varicose Veins of Pudenda.(Pelvic Congestion)
- Leucorrhoea: Acrid with Vaginal Burning.
- Discharge of Blood from genitals during stool.

184. MAGNESIA CARBONICA
(Carbonate of Magnesium)

Female:

- Sore throat before Menses appears.
- Before Menses, coryza and blocked nose.
- Menses: Too late and scanty, thick, dark with Pitch.
- Leucorrhoea of Mucus.
- Menses flow only in sleep; more.
- Profuse at night or when lying down.
- Flow ceases when walking.

185. MAGNESIA MURIATICA
(Muriate of Magnesia)

Female:

- Menses: Black, Clotted.
- Pain in back and thighs.
- Metrorrhagia; Worse at night.
- Great excitement at every period.
- Leucorrhoea with every stool and after exercise.
- Tinea Ciliaris, eruption on Face and Forehead, worse before Menses.

186. MAGNESIA PHOPHORICA
(Phosphate of Magnesia)

Female:

- Menstrual Colic
- Membranous Dysmenorrhoea
- Menses: Too early, Too stringy.
- Swelling of external parts.
- Ovarian Neuralgia.
- Vaginismus.

Abdominal Symptoms:

- Enteralgia; relieved by Pressure.
- Flatulent colic, forcing patient to bend double; relieved by rubbing. Warmth and Pressure; accompanied by Belching of Gas, which gives no relief.
- Bloated, full sensation in Abdomen; must loosen clothing, walk about and constantly pass flatus.
- Constipation in Rheumatic Subjects due to flatulence and indigestion.

187. MANGANUM ACETICUM
(Manganese Acetate)

Female:

- Derangements of Menstruation, amenorrhoea;
- Menses too early and scanty
- In anaemic subjects Flushes of heat at climacteric

188. MANGIFERA INDICA
(Mango Tree)

- One of the best general remedies for Passive Haemorrhage.
- Female
- Uterine Haemorrhage
- Varicose Veins.

189. MEDORRHINUM
(The Gonorrhoeal Virus)

Male:

- Nocturnal Emissions followed by great weakness. Impotence.
- Gleet: Whole urethra feels sore Urethritis.
- Enlarged and Painful Prostate with Frequent urging and Painful Urination.

Female:

- Intense Pruritus Menses offensive, Profuse, dark, clotted, stains difficult to wash out.
- Urinates frequently at the time of Menses.
- Sensitive spot near Uteri
- Leucorrhoea: Thin, Acrid, Excoriating, Fishy odour.
- Sycotic worts on Genitals
- Ovarian Pain: Worse Left Side or from Ovary to Ovary Sterility.
- Metrorrhagia, Intense menstrual colic.
- Breasts: Cold, sore and sensitive

190. MEDUSA
(Jelly Fish)

Female:

- Marked Action on Lacteal Glands.-Breast
- The Secretion of Milk was established after lack of it in all previous confinements.

191. MEL CUM SALE
(Honey with Salt)

Female:

- Prolapsus uteri and chronic Metritis, especially when associated with subinvolution and inflammation of the cervix.
- Feeling of soreness across the hypogastrium from ileum to ileum.
- Uterine Displacements
- Sensation as if bladder were too full.
- Pain from scarum towards Pubes.
- Pain as if in ureters.

192. MELILOTUS
(Yellow Melilot – Sweet Clover)

Female:

- Menses scanty intermit with nausea and bearing down.
- Sticking Pain in external parts.
- Dysmenorrhoea.
- Ovarian Neuralgia

194. MERCURIUS-HYDRARGYRUM
(Quicksilver)

Male:

- Vesicles and Ulcers.
- Soft Chancre
- Cold Genitals
- Prepuce irritated, Itches
- Nocturnal Emissions stained with Blood

Female:

- Menses Profuse with Abdominal Pains.
- Leucorrhoea: Excoriating, Greenish and Bloody
- Sensation of rawness in Parts.
- Stinging pain in Ovaries (Apis)
- Itching and Burning-Worse: after Urination
- Better: Washing with Cold Water
- Morning Sickness with profuse salivation
- Breast:
  Mammae Painful and Full of Milk, at the time of
  Menses.

195. MERCURIUS CORROSIVUS
(Corrosive Sublimate)

Male:

- Penis and Testes enormously swollen.
- Chancres assume phagedenic appearance.
- Gonorrhoea
- Urethra: Orifice red, swollen
- Glans: Sore and Hot.
- Discharge: Greenish, Thick.

196. MEZEREUM
(Spurge Olive)

Male:

- Enlargement of Testicles
- Violent Sexual Desire
- Gonorrhoea with Haematuria

Female:

- Menses too Frequent, soon Profuse.
- Leucorrhoea like Albumen; very corroding.

197. MILLEFOLIUM
(Achillea Millifolium)-Yarrow

Female:

- Menses early, Profuse, Protracted.
- Haemorrhage from uterus – Bright Red Fluid.
- Painful Varices during Pregnancy.

198. MITCHELLA
(Partridge - Berry)

Female:
- Cervix: dark, red, swollen.
- Dysmenorrhoea and uterine haemorrhage
- Blood: Bright Red.

199. MOMORDICA BALSAMINA
(Balsam Apple)

Female:

- Painful and Profuse menses.
- Labour – like Pains, followed by gushes of Blood
- Pain at small of Back, coming towards front of Pelvis.

200. MORPHINUM

(An Alkaloid of Opium)

Male:

- Impotency
- Pain in Right Spermatic cord. (Coxalic acid)

201. MOSCHUS
(Musk)

Male:

- Violent desire
- Involuntary Emissions
- Impotence, associated with diabetes (coca)
- Premature senility
- Nausea and vomiting after coition.

Female:

- Menses too early, too profus with disposition to faint.
- Sexual Desire with intolerable titillation in parts.
- Drawing and pushing in the direction of the genitals
- Sensation as if menses will appear.

202. MUREX
(Purple Fish)

Female:

- Consciousness of a womb.(Uterus)
- Pulsation in the neck of womb. (Uterus)
- Desire: easily excited.
- Feeling as if something was pressing on a sore spot in the Pelvis; worse: sitting.
- Pain from right side of womb to right or left Breast.
- Nymphomania.
- Least contact of parts causes violent sexual excitement.
- Sore Pain in the Uterus.
- Menses: Irregular, Profuse, frequent, large clots Feeling of Prostration, Exhaustion
- Prolapse: Enlargement of Uterus with Pelvic tenesmus and sharp Pains, extending toward Breasts. Aggravated by lying down.
- Dymenorrhoea and Chronic Endometritis, with displacement
- Must keep legs tightly crossed.
- Leucorrhoea: green or bloody, alternate with mental symptoms and aching in sacrum.
- Benign Tumours in Breasts.
- Pain in Breasts during menstrual Period.

203. MURIATICUM ACIDUM
(Muriatic Acid)

Female:

- Menses appear too soon.
- Leucorrhoea
- During menses, soreness of anus.
- Ulcer in genital.

204. MYGALE LASIODORA
(Black Cuban Spider)

Male:
- Violent erections
- Chordee (Kali Brom; Camph)

205. NAJA TRIPUDIANS
(Virus of the Cobra)

Female:

- Neuralgia of the Left Ovary; often serviceable in obscure Pain in left groin.
- Especially in Post Operative cases; seems to be drawn to heart.

206. NATRUM CARBON
(Carbonate of Sodium)

Female:
- Induration of Cervix
- Pudenda sore
- Bearing down sensation (sep; Murex)
- Heaviness; worse; sitting.
- Better: by moving
- Menses: Late, scanty, like "meat – washings".
- Leucorrhoea: discharge offensive, irritating and proceeded by colic.

207. NATRUNM CHLORATUM
(Labarraque's Solution)

Female:

- Feeling as if uterus were pushed up; on sitting down.
- Feels as if it opened and shut.
- Violent Metrorrhagia.
- Leucorrhoea and Backache.
- Passive bearing – down from heavy condition of uterus.
- Uterus is heavy, sodden with tendency to Prolapse.
- Sub involution.

208. NATRUM MURIATICUM
(Nacl = chloride of sodium)

Male:

- Emissions, even after coitus.
- Impotence with Retarded Emissions.

Female:

- Menses: Irregular; usually profuse.
- Vagina: dry.
- Leucorrhoea: Acrid, Watery.
- Bearing down Pains; worse in morning (Sep.).
- Prolapsus uteri with cutting Pain in Urethra.
- Ineffectual Labour Pains.
- Suppressed Menses.
- Hot during Menses.

209. NATRUM PHOSPHORICUM
(Phosphate of Sodium)

- Any Conditions arising from excess of Lactic acid.

Male:
- Emissions without dreams, with weakness in back and trembling in Limbs.
- Desire without erection. Gonorrhoea.

Female:
- Menses too early; Pale, Thin, Watery.
- Sterility with acid secretion from Vagina.
- Leucorrhoea: discharges creamy of honey coloured, or acid and watery.
- Sour smelling discharges from uterus.
- Morning Sickness with sour vomiting.

210. NATRUM SULPHURICUM
(Sulphate of Sodium – Glauber's salt)

Female:
- Nosebleed during Menses, which is acrid and profuse.
- Burning in pharynx during menstruation.
- Herpetic Vulvitis.
- Leucorrhoea: Yellowish – green, following gonorrhoea, discharge thick, greenish; little Pain.

211. NICCOLUM
(Metallic Nickel)

Female:

- Menses: late, scanty, with great debility and burning in eyes.
- Profuse Leucorrhoea; worse, after Urinating, worse after Menses.

212. NICCOLUM SULPHURICUM
(Sulphate of Nickle)

Female:

- Useful in climacteric disturbances.
- Dull aching in ovaries with sensation as if menses appear.
- Hot Flushes, followed by Perspiration on parts touching each other; when separated become dry.

213. NITRICUM ACIDUM
(Nitric Acid)

Male:
- Soreness and burning in glans and beneath Prepuce.
- Ulcers: burn and sting.
- Exudate: Offensive matter.

Female:
- External Parts: Sore with ulcers.
- Leucorrhoea: brown, flesh coloured, watery or stringy, offensive.
- Hair on genitals falls out. (Nat. M; Zinc)
- Uterine Haemorrhages.
- Menses: Early, Profuse, like muddy water with Pain in back, hips and thighs.
- Stitches through Vagina.
- Metrorrhagia after parturition.

214. NUX MOSCHATA
(Nutmeg)

Female:

- Uterine Haemorrhage
- Menses: Too long, dark, thick.
- Leucorrhoea: Muddy and bloody.
- Suppression with persistent fainting attacks and sleepiness.
- Variableness of Menstruation irregularities of time and quantity.
- Lypothymia
  (Lypemania = Intense Nervous Depression).

215. NUX VOMICA
(Poison - Nut)

Male:
- Easily excited desire.
- Emissions from high living.
- Bad Effects of Sexual Excess.
- Constrictive Pain in Testicles. Orchitis
- Spermatorrhoea with dreams.
- Backache, burning in spine.
- Weakness and Irritability.

Female:

- Menses: Too early, lasts too long.
- Always Irregular, Black Blood with fainting spells.
- Prolapsus Uteri
- Dysmenorrhoea with Pain in sacrum and constant urging to stool.
- Inefficient Labour Pains, extend to rectum with desire for stool and frequent Urination.
- Desire: too strong.
- Metrorrhagia with sensation as if bowels wanted to move.

216. OCIMUM CANUM
(Brazilian Alfavaca)

Male:

- Heat and Swelling of Left Testicle.

Female:

- Vulva swollen, darting Pain in Labia.
- Nipples Painful to least contact.
- Breasts feel full and tense; itching.
- Prolapsus Vaginae.

217. OLEUM ANIMALE
(Dippel's Animal Oil)

Male:

- Desire increased; ejaculation too soon.
- Pain along spermatic card to testicles.
- Testicles feel serized and pulled forcibly upward.
- Worse: Right.
- Pressure in the Perineum
- Prostatic hypertrophy.

218. OLEUM SANTALI
(Oil of Sandalwood)

Male:

- Painful Erections
- Swelling of the Prepuce.
- Thick, Yellowish, Muco – purulent discharge.
- Deep Pain in Perineum.

219. ONOSMODIUM
(False Gromwell)

Male:

- Constant Sexual Excitement.
- Psychical Impotence
- Loss of Desire
- Speedy Emissions – Deficient Erections.

Female:

- Severe Uterine Pains; bearing down Pains.
- Old Pain returns.
- Sexual Desire completely destroyed.
- Feels as if menses would appear.
- Aching in Breasts.
- Nipples itch.
- Menses too early and too prolonged.
- Soreness in uterine region.
- Leucorrhoea: Yellow, acrid, profuse.

220. OOPHORINUM
(Ovarian Extract)

Female:

- Suffering following excision of the ovaries.
- Climacteric disturbances.
- Ovarian Cysts.
- Cutaneous Disorders and Acne Rosacea.
- Prurigo.
- Menopausal Syndrome

221. OPIUM
(Dried latex of the poppy)

Female:

- Suppressed menses from fright.
- Cessation of Labour Pains with coma and twitching.
- Peurperal convulsions; Drowsiness or coma between Paroxysms.
- Threatened Abortion
- Suppression of Lochia from fright with sopor.
- Horrible Labour like Pains in Uterus; with urging to stool.

222. ORIGANUM
(Sweet Marjoram)

- Acts of Nervous System.
- Effective in excessively aroused sexual impulses.
- Affections of the Breasts. (Bufo)
- Desire for active exercise impelling her to run.

Female:

- Erotomania: Powerful lascivious impulses.
- Leucorrhoea
- Hysteria
- Lascivious ideas and dreams.

Compare:
- Ferula glauca:
  A violent sexual excitement in Women.

- Platina
- Valerina
- Cantnaris
- Hyocymus

223. OXALICUM ACIDUM
(Sorrel Acid)

Male:

- Terrible Neuralgic Pains in Spermatic Cord.
- Tesitcles feels confused and heavy.
- Seminal Vesiculitis.

224. OXYTROPIS
(Loco - Weed)

Male:
- No desire or
- No Ability to perform
- Pain in Testicles and along spermatic cord and down thighs.

225. PALLADIUM
(The Metal)

- An ovarian Remedy; Produces the symptom – complex of chronic oophoritis.
- Useful where the Parenchyma of the gland is not totally destroyed.

Female:

- Uterine Prolapse and Retroversion.
- Sub acute Pelvic Peritonitis Right – side Pain and backache.
- Menorrhagia.
- Cutting Pain in Uterus, relieved after Stool.
- Pain and Swelling in region of right ovary. Shooting or burning Pain in Pelvis and bearing down; relived by rubbing Soreness and shooting Pain from navel to Breast.
- Glairy Leucorrhoea.
- Menstrual Discharge with nursing.
- Stitches in Right Breast near nipple.

226. PARAFFINE
(Purified Paraffin)

Female:
- Menses: Too, black, abundant.
- Milky Leucorrhoea
- Nipples Painful when touched, as if sore inside.
- Stabbing Pain in Mons veneris.
- Very hot urine with burning Pains in Vulva.

227. PETROLEUM
(Crude Rock - Oil)

Male:

- Herpetic eruption on Perineum.
- Prostate inflamed and swollen.
- Itching in Urethra.

Female:

- Before Menses: Throbbing in Head. (Kreus)
- Leucorrhoea: Profuse, Albuminous.
- Genitals: Sore and Moist.
- Sensation of moisture.
- Itching and mealy coating of nipples.

228. PHOSPHORICUM ACIDUM
(Phosphoric Acid)

Male:

- Emissions at night and at stool.
- Seminal Vesiculitis (oxalic acid)
- Sexual Power deficient.
- Testicles: Tender and Swollen. Parts relax during embrace.
- Prostorrhoea, even when passing a soft stool.
- Eczema of Scrotum.
- Oedema of Prefuce and swollen glans Penis.
- Herpes preputialis.
- Sycotic excrescences. (Thuja)

Female:

- Menses: Too early and Profuse; with Pain in Liver.
- Itching
- Yellow Leucorrhoea after menses.
- Milk: scanty: flow from Breasts
- Health deteriorated from nursing.

229. PHOSPHOROUS
(Phosphorous)

Male:

- Lack of power.
- Irresistible Desire.
- Involuntary emissions with lascivious dreams.

Female:
- Metritis
- Chlorosis
- Phlebitis
- Fistulous tracks after mammary abscess.
- Slight Haemorrhage from uterus between periods.
- Menses: Too early and scanty – Not Profuse but last too long.
- Weeps before Menses.
- Stitching Pain in Mammae.
- Leucorrhoea: Profuse, smarting, corrosive instead of Menses.
- Amenorrhoea with Vicarious menses. (Bry)
- Suppuration of mammae,
- Burning, watery, offensive discharge.
- Nymphomania
- Uterine Polyps.

230. PHYSOSTIGMA
(Calabar bean)

Female:

- Irregular Menstruation with Palpitation.
- Congestion of Eyes.
- Rigid Muscles.

231. PHYTOLACCA
(Poke -Root)

Male:
- Painful Induration of Testicles.
- Shooting along Perineum to Penis.

Female:
- Mastitis; mamme hard and very sensitive.
- Tumours of the Breast with enlarged axillary glands.
- Cancer of Breasts.
- Breast is hard, Painful and of Purple hue.
- Mammary Abscess.
- When child nurses, Pain goes from nipple to all over body.
- Cracks and small ulcers about nipples.
- Irritable breasts, before and during menses.
- Galactarrhoea.
- Menses: Too copious and too frequent.
- Ovarian Neuralgia of Right side.

232. PICRICUM ACIDUM
(Picric acid - Trinitrophenol)

Male:

- Emissions Profuse followed by great exhaustion;
- Without sensual dream.
- Priapism – Satyriasis.
- Hard erections with Pain in testicles and upward in the cord.
- Prostatic Hypertrophy; especially in cases not too far advanced.

Female:

- Pain in Left Ovary and Leucorrhoea before menstruation.
- Pruritus vulvae.

233. PITUITARY GLAND

- Having a superior control over the growth and development of the sexual organs.
- Uterine Inertia.
- Second stage of Labour where the Ext. OS is fully dilated

234. PLATINA

Female:

- Parts Hyper sensitive.
- Tingling internally and externally.
- Ovaries: sensitive and burn.
- Menses: Too early, too profuse, dark – clotted with spasm and painful bearing down.
- Chilliness and sensitiveness of parts.
- "Vaginismus"
- Nymphomania
- Excessive sexual development:
- Vaginismus.
- Pruritis vulvae.
- Ovaritis with Sterility.
- Abnormal sexual appetite and Melancholia

235. PLUMBUM METALLICUM
(Lead)

Male:

- Loss of Sexual Power. Testicles drawn up, feel constricted.

Female:

- "Vaginismus" with emaciation and constipation.
- Induration of Mammary Glands.
- Vulva and Vagina hypersensitive. Stitches and burning Pain in Breasts. Tendency to Abortion.
- Menorrhagia with sensation of string pulling from Abdomen to back. Disposition to Yawn and Stretch.

236. PODOPHYLLUM
(May - Apple)

Female:

- Pains in Uterus and Right Ovary; with shifting noises along ascending colon.
- Suppressed menses with Pelvic tenesmus.
- Prolapsed uteri, especially after parturition.
- Haemorrhoids with prolapsus ani during pregnancy.
- Prolapsus from over lifting or
- straining during Pregnancy

237. POLYGONUM PUNCTATUM
(Smart Weed)

Female:

- Metrorrhagia.
- Amenorrhoea in young girls.
- Varicosis.
- Aching pain in hips and loins.
- Sensation as if hips were being drawn together.
- Sensation of weight and tension with in Pelvia.
- Shooting Pains through Breasts.
- Amenorrhoea.

238. PSORINUM
(Scabies Vesicle)

Female:

- Leucorrhoea: foetid, lumpy with much backache and debility.
- Mammae: Swollen and Painful
- Pimples: Oozing an acrid fluid that burns and excoriates the glands.

239. PULEX IRRITANS
(Common Flea)

Female:

- Menses: Delayed.
- Increased flow of Saliva during menses.
- Intense burning in Vagina.
- Leucorrhoea: Profuse, foul, staining a Greenish yellow.
- Stains of menses and Leucorrhoea very hard to wash out.
- Backache.

240. PULSATILLA
(Wind Flower)

- Pre-eminently a female remedy.
- Consti: Mild, Gentle, Yielding disposition,
- Sad, crying readily, weeps when talking, changeable, contradictory seeking open air.

Male:

- Orchitis; Pain from abdomen to testicles.
- Thick, yellow discharge from Urethra.
- Late Stage of Gonorrhoea.
- Stricture: Urine passed only in drops and stream interrupted. (Clemat)
- Acute Prostatitis
- Pain and Tenesmus in Urinating,
- Worse lying on back.

Female:

- Amenorrhoea: Suppressed menses from wet feet.
- Nervous debility or Chlorosis.
- Menses: Tardy menses; too late, scanty, thick, dark, clotted, changeable, intermittent.
- Chilliness, nausea, downward pressure, Painful, flow intermits.
- Leucorrhoea: Acrid, burning, and creamy.
- Pain in Back, Tired feeling.
- Diarrhoea during or after menses.

241. PYROGENIUM
(Artificial Sepsin)

Female:

- Puerperal peritonitis, with extreme fetor.
- Septicaemia following abortions.
- Menses horribly offensive.
- Uterine Haemorrhage.
- Fever at each menstrual period, consequent upon latent pelvic inflammation.
- Septic puerperal infection.
- Pelvic calculitis
- Inflammatory exudate.
- Post – operative cases with overwhelming sepsis.

242. RADIUM
(Radium Bromide)

Female:

- Pruritus vulvae.
- Delayed and irregular menstruation and Backache.
- Aching Pains in abdomen Over Pubes when flow comes on.
- Right Breast: Sore, Relieved by Hard Rubbing.

243. RAPHANUS
(Black Garden Radish)

Female:

- Nervous irritation of Genitals.
- Menses very Profuse and Long – lasting.
- Nymphomania with aversion to her own sex.
- Aversion to children
- Sexual Insomnia.

244. RHODODENDRON
(Snow - Rose)

Male:

- Testicles, worse on left side.
- Swollen, Painful, drawn-up.
- Orchitis: Glands feel crushed.
- Induration and swelling of testes after Gonorrhoea.
- Hydrocele.

245. RHUS TOXICODENDRON
(Poison - Ivy)

Male:

- Swelling of Glands and Prepuce, dark, Red, Erysepelatous.
- Scrotum: Thick, Swollen, Oedematous.
- Itching intense.

Female:

- Swelling, with intense itching of vulva.
- Pelvic articulation stiff when beginning to move.
- Menses: early profus and prolonged, acrid.
- Lochia: Thin, Protracted, offensive, diminished with shooting upwards in vagina.

246. ROBINIA

(Yellow Locust)

Female:

- Nymphomania
- Acrid, foetid leucorrhoea
- Discharge of Blood between menstrual Periods.
- Herpes on vagina and vulvae.

247. SABADILLA
(Asagraea Officinalis – Cevadilla Seed)

Female:
- Menses: Too late; come by fits and starts.
- Intermit (Kreos, Puls).
- Due to transient and localized congestion in Uterus – alternating with chronic anaemic state.

248. SABAL SERRULATA
(Saw Palmetto)

Male:

- Prostatic Troubles: enlargement.
- Discharge of Prostatic fluid.
- Wasting of testes and loss of Sexual Power.
- Coitus Painful at the time of emissions.
- Sexual Neurotics.
- Organs feel cold.

Female:

- Ovaries tender and enlarged.
- Breasts shrivel. (Iod, Kali. iod)
- Young Female neurotics.
- Suppressed or Perverted sexual Inclination

249. SABINA
(Savine)

Male:

- Inflammatory gonorrhoea, with Pus-like discharge
- Sycotic excrescences.
- Burning, sore Pain in glans.
- Prepuce Painful with difficulty in retracting it.

Female:

- Menses Profuse, bright.
- Uterine Pains extend into thighs.
- Threatened Miscarriage.
- Sexual desire increased.
- Leucorrhoea after menses: corrosive, Offensive.
- Discharge of blood between periods with sexual excitement. (Ambr.)
- Retained Placenta; intense after – Pains.
- Menorrhagia in women who aborted readily.
- Inflammation of ovaries and uterus after abortion.
- Promotes expulsion of moles from uterus (Cantharis)
- Pain from sacrum to pubes and from below upwards shooting up the vagina.
- Haemorrhage: partly clotted: Worse, from least motion.
- Atony of Uterus.

250. SALIX NIGRA
(Black - Willow)

Female:

- Before and during menses much nervous disturbances.
- Pain in Ovaries.
- Difficult Menstruation.
- Ovarian Congestion and Neuralgia.
- Menorrhagia
- Bleeding with Uterine fibroid.
- Nymphomania.

251. SANGUINARIA
(Blood Root)

Female:

- Leucorrhoea: foetid, corrosive
- Menses: Offensive, Profuse.
- Soreness of Breasts.
- Uterine Polypii
- Before Menses: Itching of axillae.
- Climacteric disorders.

252. SANICULA (Aqua)

The Water of Sanicula Springs - Ottawa.

Female:

- Bearing down, as if contents of Pelvis would escape. Better by Rest.
- Desire to support parts.
- Soreness of Uterus.
- Leucorrhoea with odour of fish -brine or old cheese (Hepar)
- Vagina feels large.

253. SARSAPARILLA
(Smilax)

Male:

- Bloody seminal Emissions. Intolerable stench on genitals. Herpetic eruptions on genitals.
- Itching on scrotum and Perineum. Syphilis; squamous eruptions and bone pains.

Female:
- Nipples small, withered, retracted.
- Before menstruation, - Itching and Humid
- Eruptions on forehead.
- Menses: Late and Scanty
- Moist eruptions in Right Groin before Menses.

254. SECALE CORNUTUM
(Ergot) claviceps purpurea

Female:
- Menstrual colic, with coldness and intolerance of heat.
- Passive Haemorrhages in feeble, cachectic women.
- Burning pain in uterus.
- Brownish, offensive leucorrhoea.
- Menses: Irregular, copious, dark. Continuous oozing of watery blood until next period.
- Threatened Abortion about the Third Month.
- During labour: No expulsive action, though everything is relaxed.
- After Pains.
- Suppression of milk.
- Breasts do not fill properly.
- Dark, offensive lochia.
- Puerperal fever; putrid discharges.
- Tympanitis
- Coldness
- Suppressed Urine.

255. SELENIUM
(The Element-Selenium)

Male:

- Dribbling of semen during sleep.
- Dribbling of Prostatic fluid.
- Irritability after coitus.
- Loss of sexual power, with lascivious fancies.
- Increases desire, decreases ability.
- Semen: Thin and Odourless
- Sexual Neureasthenia.
- On attempting coition, Penis relaxes.
- Hydrocele.

256. SENECIO AUREUS
(Golden Ragwort)

Male:
- Lascivious dreams with involuntary emissions.
- Prostate enlarged.
- Dull, heavy Pain in spermatic cord, extending to testicles.

Female:
- Menses Retarded, suppressed.
- Functional Amenorrhoea of young girls with Backache. Before menses, inflammatory condition of Throat, chest and Bladder, after flow starts, all these, improves
- Anaemic dysmenorrhoea with urinary disturbances.
- Premature and too profuse menses.

257. SEPIA
(Inky Juice of Cuttle Fish)

Sepia acts best on Brunettes.

Male:
- Organs Cold.
- Offensive Perspiration
- Gleet, Discharge from Urethra –only during night.
- No Pain
- Condylomata- surround the head of penis.
- Complains from Coition.

Female:
- Pelvic Organs relaxed.
- Bearing down sensation as if everything would escape from vulva.
- Must cross her legs/ limbs to prevent protrusion.
- Leucorrhoea: Yellow, Greenish with much itching.
- Menses: Too late and scanty, Irregular,
- Early and profuse, Sharp, clutching pains
- Violent stitches upwards in the vagina, from uterus to Umbilicus.
- Prolapse of Uterus
- Prolapse of Vagina
- Vagina: painful especially on Coition.
- Morning Sickness.

258. SILICEA
(Silica - Pure Flint)

Male:
- Burning and soreness of Genitals with eruptions on inner surface of thighs.
- Chronic Gonorrhoea, with thick, foetid discharge.
- Elephantiasis of scrotum.
- Sexual Erythism
- Nocturnal Emissions.
- Hydrocele.

Female:

- A milky acrid Leucorrhoea during Urination.
- Itching of Vulva and Vagina-Very Sensitive.
- Discharge of Blood between Menstrual Periods.
- Increased Menses, with paroxysms of icy coldness over whole body.
- Nipples: Very sore, Ulcerated easily, Drawn in (Retracted)
- Fistulous Ulceration of Breast (Phos)
- Abscess of Labia
- Discharge of blood from vagina, every time child is nursed.
- Vaginal Cysts (Lyco, Puls, Rhodo)
- Hard Lumps in Breasts (Conium)

259. SOLIDAGO VIRGA
(Golden Rod)

Female:
- Uterine Enlargement
- Organs pressed down upon the Bladder.
- Fibroid Tumours.

260. SPIRANTHES
(Lady's Tresses)

It has been used for Milk-Flow in nursing women.

Female:
- Pruritus : Vulvae red, swollen
- Dryness and Burning in Vagina
- Burning pain in vagina during coition
- Leucorrhoea: Bloody

261. SPONGIA TOSTA
(Roasted Sponge)

Male:

- Swelling of spermatic cord and testicles with pain and tenderness.
- Orchitis.
- Epididymitis
- Heat in Parts.

Female:

- Before Menses, pain in Sacrum, Hunger and Palpitation.
- During Menses, wakes with suffocative spells.
- Amenorrhoea with Asthma.

262. STANNUM
(Tin)

Female:

- Bearing Down sensation
- Prolapsus with weak, sinking feeling in stomach (Sep)
- Menses: Early and Profuse
- Pain in vagina: Upward and Backward to Spine
- Leucorrhoea with great debility.

263. STAPHYSAGRIA
(Stavesacre)

Male:

- Especially after self abuse, Persistent dwelling on sexual subjects
- Spermatorrhoea with sunken features.
- Guilty Look.
- Emissions with backache and weakness.
- Sexual Neurasthenia.
- Dyspnoea after coition.

264. STICTA
(Lungwort)

Female:
- Scanty Flow of Milk.

265. STRAMONIUM
(Thorn Apple)

Male:

- Sexual Erythism with indecent speech and action.
- Hand constantly keeps on Genitals.

Female:

- Metrorrhagia with Loquacity, Singing, Praying
- Puerperal Mania with characteristic Mental Symptoms and profuse sweating.
- Convulsions after Labour.

266. STROPHANTHUS HISPIDUS
(Kombe-Seed)

Female:
- Menorrhagia
- Uterine Haemorrhage
- Uterus heavily congested
- Aching pains through Hips.

267. STRYCHNINUM
(Alkaloid of Nux Vomica)

Female:

- Desire for coitus
    (Canth. Camph. Fl.acid, Lach. Phos.Plat.)
- Any touch on body excites a voluptuous sensation.

268. SULPHUR
(Sublimated Sulphur)

Male:
- Stitches in Penis.
- Involuntary Emissions.
- Itching of Genitals when going to bed.
  (Nocturnal Pruritus)
- Organs: Cold, Relaxed and Powerless.

Female:
- Pudenda itches, Vagina burns.
- Much offensive perspiration
- Menses: Too late, too Short, Scanty and Difficult, Thick, Black, Acrid,
- Making parts sore.
- Menses preceded by headache, or
- Menses suddenly stopped.
- Leucorrhoea: Burning, Excoriating
- Nipples: Cracked, Smart and Burns.

269. SULPHURICUM ACIDUM
(Sulphuric Acid)

Female:
- Menstruation early and profuse.
- Erosion of Cervix in the aged.
- Easily Bleeding, Bleeding on Touch.
- Acrid, Burning Leucorrhoea, often of bloody mucus.

270. SUMBUL-FERULA SUMBUL
(Musk-Root)

Female:
- Ovarian Neuralgia
- Abdomen: Full,
- Distended
- Painful
- Climacteric Flushes, Hot flushes

271. SYPHILINUM

Female:

- Ulcers on Labia
- Leucorrhoea: Profuse, Thin, Watery, Acrid with sharp knife like pain ovaries.

272. TINACETUM VULGARE
(Tansy)

Female:
- Dysmenorrhoea with bearing down pains,
- Tenderness, drawing in groins
- Menses: Suppressed
- Menses: Later...Profuse.

273. TARENTULA HISPANIA
(Spanish Spider)

Male:
- Sexual Excitement
- Lasciviousness reaching almost to Insanity.
- Seminal Emissions.

Female:
- Vulvae dry and Hot with much itching.
- Profuse menstruation, with frequent Erotic spasms.
- Pruritus Vulvae.
- Nymphomania
- Dysmenorrhoea with very sensitive ovaries.

274. TEREBENTHINA
(Turpentine)

Female:
- Intense burning in Uterine Region.
- Metritis
- Puerperal Parotinitis
- Metrorrhagia with burning in Uterus

275. THASPIUM AUREUM-ZIZIA

(Meadow Parsnip)

Male:

- Great Lassitude following coitus
- Sexual power increased.

Female:

- Intermittent Neuralgia : Left Ovary
- Acrid, Profuse Leucorrhoea with retarded menses.

276. THEA
(Tea)

Female:
- Soreness and Tenderness in Ovaries.

277. THIOSINAMINU - RHODALLIN
(A chemical derived from oil of Mustard)

A Resolvent: Externally and internally for dissolving Scar tissues.

- Tumours
- Enlarged Glands
- Lumps
- Strictures
- Adhesions

278. THLASPI BURSA PASTORIS CAPSELLA
(Shepherd`s Purse)

Male:
- Spermatic cord sensitive to concussion of walking or riding.

Female:

- Metrorrhagia: Too frequent and copious menses
- Haemorrhage with violent uterine colic
- Every alternate period very profuse.
- Leucorrhoea: before and after menses. which is
- Bloody, dark, offensive, stains indelibly
- Sore pain in uterus on rising.
- Scarcely recovers from one period before another begins.

279. THUJA
(Arbor Vitae)

Male:

- Inflammation of prepuce and Glans
- Pain in penis – Balanitis
- Gonorrhoea
- Gonorrhoeal Rheumatism
- Chronic induration of Testicles
- Pain and burning felt near neck of Urinary Bladder,
- With frequent and urgent desire to urinate
- Prostatic Enlargement (Ferr.Pic, Thiosin, Iod, Sabal)

Female:

- Vagina very sensitive (Berb, Kreos, Lyssin)
- Warty excrescences on vulva and perineum
- Leucorrhoea: Profuse, Thick, Greenish
- Severe pain: Left Ovary and Left Inguinal Region
- Menses: scanty, retarded.
- Polyp: Fleshy excrescence
- Ovaritis: worse: Left Side: at every menstrual period.
- Profuse Perspiration before menses.

280. THYMOL
(Thyme Camphor)

Male:
- Profuse, nightly seminal emissions with lascivious dreams of a perverted character
- Priapism
- Urinary Burning and subsequent dribbling of Urine.
- Polyuria
- Urates increased
- Phosphates decreased.

281. TILIA EUROPA
(Linden)

Female:
- Intense sore feeling about uterus.
- Bearing down with hot sweat but without relief
- Leucorrhoea: Much Slimy when walking
- Soreness and Redness of external genitals
- Pelvic Inflammation
- Tympanitis
- Abdominal Tenderness and hot sweat, which does not relieve.

282. TRIBULUS TERRESTRIS
(Ikshugandha)

An East Indian drug useful in debilitated state of the Sexual Organs, as expressed in seminal weakness, ready emissions and impoverished Semen.

- Prostatitis
- Calculous affection
- Sexual Neurasthenia
- It meets the Auto-Traumatism of Masturbation, correcting the emissions and spermatorrhoea.
- Partial Impotence caused by overindulgence of advancing age.

283. TRILLIUM PENDULUM
(White beth root)

Female:

- Uterine Haemorrhages with sensation as…
  Though Back and Hips were falling to pieces and
  feels better by tight bandages
- Gushing of bright blood on least movement
- Haemorrhage from Fibroids.
- Prolapse with great bearing down.
- Leucorrhoea: Copious, Yellow, and Stringy.
- Metrorrhagia at Climecteric.
- Lochia: suddenly becomes sanguineous
- Dribbling of urine after Labour.

284. TUBERCULINUM

(A nucleo-protein, a nosode from Tubercular Abscess)

Female:
- Benign Mammary Tumours.
- Menses: Too early, Too Profuse, And Long Lasting.
- Dysmenorrhoea
- Pain increases with the establishment of Flow.

285. TURNERA—DAMIANA

Male:

- Very useful in Sexual Neurasthenia.
- Impotency.
- Sexual debility from nervous prostration.
- Incontinence in old people.
- Chronic Prostatic Discharge.

Female:

- Aids the establishment of Normal Menstrual Flow in young girls.
- Frigidity of Female

286. TUSSILAGO PETASITES
(Butter burr)

Male:

- Gonorrhoea: Yellowish, Thick discharge.
- Erections with Urethral crawling.
- Pain in Spermatic cord.

287. UPAS TIENTE
(Upas tree - Antiaris Toxicaria)

Male:
- Desire increased, with loss of power.
- Dull backache, as after excessive coitus.

288. URANIUM NITRATE
(Nitrate of Uranium)

Male:
- Complete Impotency with nocturnal emissions.
- Organs cold, Relaxed, Sweaty.

289. URTICA URENUS

(Stinging nettle)

Male:

- Itching of scrotum, keeps him awake.
- Scrotum: Swollen.

Female:

- Diminished secretion of Milk.
- Uterine Haemorrhage
- Acid and Excoriating Leucorrhoea
- Pruritus Vulvae with stinging, itching and oedema.
- Arrests flow of Milk after weaning.
- Excessive swelling of breasts.

290. USTILIGO MAYDIS
(Corn smut)

- Flabby condition of Uterus. Haemorrhage.
- Congestion of various parts, especially at Climacteric.
- Crusta Lactea.

Male:

- Uncontrollable Masturbation.
- Spermatorrhoea with Erotic Fancies and Amorous Dreams.
- Emissions with irresistible tendency to masturbation.
- Dull pain in Lumbar Region with great despondency and mental irritability.

Female:

- Vicarious Menstruation.
- Ovaries: Burn, Pain and Swell.
- Profuse menses after miscarriage.
- Discharge of –bright red, partly clotted Blood after slightest provocation.
- Menorrhagia after Climaxis.
- Oozing of dark blood, clotted, forming long black string.
- Uterus: Hypertrophied. Cervix bleeds easily.
- Post partum Haemorrhage.
- Profuse Lochia.

291. VALARINA
(Valerian)

Female:
- Hysteria, over sensitiveness, Nervous Affections.
- Hysterical Flatulency.
- Menses: Late and Scanty.

292. VERATRUM ALBUM
(White Hellebore)

Female:

- Menses: Too Early, Profuse and Exhausting.
- Dysmenorrhoea with coldness, purging and cold sweat.
- Faints from least exertion.
- Sexual Mania preceded by menses.

293. VERATRUM VIRIDE
(White American Hellebore)

Female:
- Rigid Os
- Purpureal Fever.
- Suppressed Menstruation with congestion to head.
- Menstrual Colic before the appearance of the discharge with strangury.

294. VESPA CRABRO
(Live Wasp)

Female:

- Menstruation, preceded by depression, pain, pressure and constipation.
- Left Ovary markedly affected with frequent burning micturition.
- Sacral Pains extending up back.
- Erosion around External Os.

295. VIBURNUM OPULUS
(High Cranberry)

- Cramps: Colicky pains in Pelvic Organs.
- Super Conscious of internal sexual organs.
- Often prevents miscarriage.
- False Labour Pains.
- Spasmodic and congestive affections, dependent upon ovarian or uterine region.

Female:

- Menses too late, scanty, lasting a few hours.
- Offensive in odour with crimpy pains. Cramps extend down thighs.
- Bearing down pains before.
- Ovarian region feels heavy and congested.
- Aching in sacrum and pubes, with pain in Anterior muscle of thighs.
- Spasmodic and Membranous Dysmenorrhoea.
- Leucorrhoea: Excoriating, Smarting and Itching of Genitals
- Faint on attempting to sit up.
- Frequent and Early, Very Early Miscarriage, causing Sterility.
- Pains from back to Loins and Womb.
- Worse: Early Morning.

296. VINCA MINOR
(Lesser Periwinkle)

Female:
- Excessive Menstruation with great weakness.
- Passive Uterine Haemorrhage.
- Menorrhagia, Continuous Flow particularly at Climacteric.
- Haemorrhages from Fibroids.

297. VIOLA TRICOLOR
(Pansy)

Male:
- Swelling of prepuce, burning in Glans.
- Itching.
- Involuntary Seminal Emissions at stool.

298. VISCUM ALBUM
(Mistletoe)

Female:
- Haemorrhage, with pain,
- Blood partly clotted and bright red.
- Climacteric Complains.
- Pain from Sacrum in to pelvis, with tearing, shooting pains, from above downwards.
- Retained Placenta.
- Chronic Endometritis.
- Metrorrhagia
- Ovaralgia, especially Left.

299. WYTHIA
(Poison weed)

Female:

- Neuralgic Dysmenorrhoea
- Menses too early and painful.
- Ovarian Neuralgia with pain in Loin and Lower Abdomen.
- Worse: Left side, extending down the thighs, along Genito-crural nerve.
- Neuralgic Dysmenorrhoea, with neuralgic headaches.
- Pain in Back and down the Legs.
- Menses: Thick, almost black. After Pains.
- Leucorrhoea at the time of menses.
- Neurasthenic patients who are thin, emaciated, poor assimilation with Insomnia and occipital headache.

300. XEROPHYLLUM
(Tamalpais Lilly, Basket Grass Flower)

Female:
- Bearing Down sensation.
- Vulva inflamed with furious itching.
- Increased Sexual Desire with ovarian and uterine pains.
- Leucorrhoea.

301. X-RAY
(Vial Containing Alcohol exposed to X-Ray)

- Has property of stimulating Cellular Metabolism.
- Arouses Reactive Vitality, Mentally and Physically.
- Its Homeopathic action is centrifugal.
- Brings suppressed symptoms to the periphery.

Male:
- Lewd dreams.
- Sexual Desire lost.
- Re-establishes suppressed Gonorrhoea

302. YOHIMBINUM
(Coryanthe Yohimbe)

Male:
- Excites Sexual organs.
- Acts on central nervous system.
- An Aphrodisiac.
- Congestive conditions of sexual organs.
- Strong and Lasting Erections.
- Neurasthenic Impotence.

Female:
- Causes Hyperaemia of the milk glands and stimulates the function of Lactation.
- Menorrhagia.

303. ZINCUM METALLICUM
(Zinc)

Male:

- Testicles swelled, drawn up.
- Erections violent.
- Emissions with Hypochondriasis.
- Falling of pubic hair.
- Drawing in Testicles up to spermatic cord.

Female:

- Ovarian pain, especially Left.
- Can't keep still.
- Nymphomania of lying-in women.
- Menses: Too late, Suppressed.
- Menses: Flow more at Night.
- Lochia: Suppressed.
- Breasts painful, Nipples sore.
- All complains are better during Menses.
- All the Female Symptoms are associated with...
  - Restlessness
  - Depression
  - Coldness
  - Spinal Tenderness....and Restless Fever.
  - Dry cough before and during menses.

304. ZINCUM VALERIANUM
(Valerinate of zinc)

Neuralgia

Female:
- Ovaralgia
- Pain shoots down limbs, even to foot.

305. ZINZIBER
(Ginger)

- Debility in Sexual system.

Male:
- Itching of prepuce.
- Sexual Desire: Excited
- Painful Erections and Emissions